THE BUM BACK BOOK

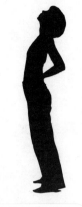

THE
BUM
BACK
BOOK

ACUPRESSURE SELF HELP BACK CARE
FOR RELIEVING TENSION AND PAIN

MICHAEL REED GACH
Foreword by GAIL MONICA DUBINSKY, M.D.

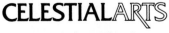
CELESTIALARTS

Berkeley, California

NOTICE: This book contains certain exercises and procedures to aid in preventing and relieving back tensions. It does not make any specific medical recommendations. Any person experiencing a back problem should consult with a holistic physician prior to engaging in any of the exercises or procedures described herein.

Celestial Arts
P.O. Box 7327
Berkeley, CA 94707

Printed in the United States of America

Library of Congress Catalog Card Number 83-71044
ISBN: 0-89087-417-4

Acknowledgments

THE TALENT and skills of seven women have improved the quality of *The Bum Back Book*. Connie Cronin's creative ideas sparked me to write the book and her input has been valuable from beginning to end. Gail Dubinsky, M.D. wrote the material on the causes of back problems and was my medical advisor. Ana Vertel and Carolyn Marco edited the manuscript several times and Ana took most of the photographs. Jenny Josephian did an outstanding job of editing and reorganizing this material into a comprehensive whole. Lynda Silva and Patricia Molino spent hours of hard work on the graphic production of the book.

I want to acknowledge Patrick Miller of *Words & Type* who typeset the manuscript and advised me on the book design. Greg Hastings, Elizabeth Delphey, Thomas Morris, Nancy Austin, Jane Brundage, Karen Keating and Judith Jang contributed their professional advice on the graphic arts. Christel Busch, R.N. and Judith Jang did the anatomical drawings. I also want to thank Andrew Partos and James Lerager for their photography, Lynda Silva and Judith Jang contributed special graphic art techniques and Bill Schwab shot the photography for the cover. My dear friends Josh Baran and Kim Marienthal gave me support and guidance. Gary Isaacson named *The Bum Back Book* and has played a major role in its success.

Credit for the high quality of this book goes to all the people mentioned above. I only provided the material for the book and coordinated these tremendous talents.

—*Michael Reed Gach*

Table of Contents

FOREWORD

Approximately 80% of all people are afflicted with significant back pain at least once during their lives. After heart conditions and arthritis, back problems are the third leading cause of limited physical activity and the most common cause of occupational disability, keeping seven million people a day off work in the U.S. In fact, up to one-third of all workers' compensation claims are for back pain or injuries incurred by or aggravated on the job.

Self Care:
The Essential Key to Optimum Health

It is my firm belief that *everybody* (physical condition permitting) should incorporate *at least* fifteen minutes of Acu-Yoga stretching exercises into their daily routine, with a proper balance of spinal movement in all directions (as outlined in this book). In addition, everybody should be aware of and avoid whenever possible postural positions that are harmful to the back, particularly improper sitting, bending, and lifting. Applying these two preventative principles alone would alleviate a phenomenal number of backaches and pains and make any concurrent professional treatments more effective. Judging from the number of patients I see in clinics and emergency rooms who have little or no concept of how they can help themselves by the simplest of stretches, exercises or relaxation techniques, the need for a book such as this is very great indeed!

What makes *The Bum Back Book* even more special is its orientation toward the ancient Eastern concepts of health maintenance. Now more than ever, the philosophies and practices of Oriental healing are being studied and applied in the United States and other Western nations, just as Western techniques are being utilized by and adapted to modern Chinese and Japanese health care systems. Although so far it has been difficult to "prove" by "scientific" means why Acupressure and Shiatsu health maintenance are so effective for relieving pain and tension, everybody can experience the healing benefits of the power of touch. The basic exercises, Acupressure points, principles and techniques, as outlined in the following pages, can be easily learned and applied by anyone interested in furthering the well-being of themselves, their friends, and their family. Using these practical tools in your daily life will not only help relieve your back problems, but also increase your possibility of achieving optimum health.

GAIL MONICA DUBINSKY M.D.

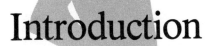

Introduction

The Bum Back Book gives practical techniques for helping yourself and others release back tension and relieve pain. **Acu-Yoga**, an integration of Acupressure* and yoga postures, will be the main technique used for self help. **Shiatsu**, a Japanese form of massage therapy that utilizes finger (*shi*) pressure (*atsu*) on Acupressure points will be used to relieve back tension on others. This book presents many alternative methods such as breathing techniques, visualizations, meditations, and Reflexology.

The stretching, strengthening and balancing techniques of these practices have been used for thousands of years in the Orient to keep people well. Through the use of movements, postures and massage techniques that stretch the muscles and meridians and press certain points, Shiatsu and Acu-Yoga effectively release tensions and restore the natural harmony of the body.

Acupressure and Acu-Yoga increase your awareness of your posture, of how you hold your body at all times and in all situations. As you cultivate this awareness, you can begin to work at correcting your poor postural habits. As your awareness grows, you will recognize and thus be able to correct any slumped-over or twisted positions sooner than you otherwise would. This body awareness helps you to perceive an imbalance at an early stage of its development, so that you can do something about it before it grows into a larger problem.

When one area of the back is stiff the body automatically compensates by taking pressure off that area and shifting it to another in order to relieve the strain and effort that can be caused even by common everyday movements. This, of course, shifts an extra burden to another area of the back, compounding the problem. It's important to work on back pain as soon as you notice it, rather than "trying to ignore it" until it becomes so bad that the ache or pain becomes an unavoidable center of attention.

Acupressure

Acupressure works to relax muscular tension and balance the vital forces of the body through a system of points and meridians. The points are places that have a high electrical conductivity on the surface of the skin, where the forces can be manipulated and balanced. The meridians† are pathways along which the energy flows from point to point.

---

*Both Acupressure and Acupuncture are based on the same principles, meridians and points. Acupuncture uses needles to stimulate points whereas Acupressure uses finger pressure and the power of human touch.

†Please refer to Glossary, page 124, for description of each individual meridian.

Locating Acupressure Points

Many of the primary Acupressure points are located in muscular areas. Tension often accumulates around these points. Sometimes the area is quite large and covers major muscles, particularly around the back and shoulders. You can actually locate a point by feeling for this tension, which is usually in the form of a *tight muscular band, cord,* or *knot* surrounding the point.

Often a point is indicated by some degree of soreness upon pressure. Look for a spot approximately the size of a dime located near the center of tight areas. It will feel sore when pressure is applied. If there is extreme (or an increase in) sensitivity or pain, gradually decrease the pressure until a balance is achieved between pain and pleasure.

Soreness upon pressure or tension surrounding a point indicates a blockage. Several minutes of firm finger pressure on these specific points strongly helps to release blockages and rebalance the body.

Sometimes an Acupressure point is not sore when pressed or is not found in an area where muscular tension forms. Many of these Acupressure points are located in anatomically important locations, such as joints or bone depressions. In this case, there will usually be a small dip or hollow in which the point can be found.

How Acupressure Works To Relieve Pain

Several theories exist to explain how Acupressure relieves pain. One explanation is the "pain-gateway" theory. This theory suggests that the transmission of pain impulses can be altered by a gating mechanism in the pain signaling system. An open gate results in pain; a partially open gate, less intense pain; and a closed gate, no pain. Acupuncture needles and Acupressure produce a mild, fairly painless stimulation which causes the gates to close so that painful sensations cannot pass through the spinal cord to the brain.*

A second theory suggests that Acupressure and Acupuncture stimulate the pituitary gland to release endorphins, which inhibit pain receptors from connecting. Endorphins, the body's natural neural-chemicals, have an effect similar to a narcotic, blocking the sensation of pain.

Independent of the various scientific theories which hope to explain how it works, Acupressure releases muscular tension and creates an "alpha-wave" response in the brain. This deep relaxation increases circulation, which removes toxins from the body and promotes a sense of general well-being.

---

*Acupuncture Therapy—Current Chinese Practice, Leng T. Tan, Margaret Y. C. Tan and Ilsa Veith, Copyright 1973 by Temple University, pub. 1973, pg. 9.

Back disorders occur almost as frequently among people with sedentary lives as among those who regularly engage in heavy physical labor. In fact, back problems are one of the most common ailments in our society. Almost everyone has experienced stiffness, tension, or pain in some part of their back, and many people suffer from it for years.

Causes of Back Pain

There are many elements which may contribute to back pain. Often, we try to isolate and blame one thing for causing us pain when, in fact, our pain may be due to a combination of causes. It is best to recognize all contributing factors so that their individual and combined effects can be understood. Consider a few of the following possibilities:

Weak Musculature: Just as the bone structure in the body acts as a support frame for the muscles, the musculature also serves to give necessary reinforcement to the bones, much like the components of a suspension bridge act on one another to hold steady the bridge as a whole. The spinal column functions very much like a bridge, connecting our upper and lower halves. When the upper body muscles, specifically those of the stomach and lower back do not support the spine-bridge, it will sag from its correct curvature, with resultant pain. Instinctively, we will try to return the spinal column to its proper position by tensing the muscles. This compensation tends to strain the back. Good muscle tone is needed for proper support. Strengthening exercises for these muscles, combined with certain yoga postures for lengthening the spine, can erase the strain and pressure in your back and improve your posture naturally.

Poor Posture: In order to maintain a strong back, free of chronic pain, the spine must remain flexible and be able to move in all directions. Currently, more and more therapists are recognizing that a large percentage of back pain is caused by a loss of flexibility and normal curve in the lower back. Constriction of the surrounding musculature, resulting from accidents or from deep-seated emotional holding, can pull the spine out of normal alignment. Often, though, the curve of the lower back reverses simply because of poor postural habits. This includes spending many hours slumped in poorly designed chairs or sleeping on non-supportive mattresses. Habitual tension and improper standing posture can also exaggerate the lower curve, producing a sway back and protruding abdomen. Any habitual deviation from a slight S curve, whether a reversal or an exaggeration, can create chronic pain. Keep in mind that movement, flexibility and diversity of posture are all important in maintaining the health of your back.

Structural Problems: Another source of back pain is structural problems of the spine. These include scoliosis (a lateral curvature and rotation of the spine), defects within the vertebrae themselves, decreased flexibility and range of motion of the various spinal joints, and misalignments—minute rotations of one vertebrae relative to its neighbor or to the attached ribs.

Arthritis: Arthritic changes can give rise to bone spurs in the spine. These spurs occur especially in the cervical (neck) vertebrae, often causing neck pain which radiates to the shoulder, scapular (shoulder blade) region, arm or hands.

Problems with Internal Organs: Both Western and Oriental medical systems relate malfunctioning of the internal organs to pain in the back. Both authorities state that this occurs via nerve connections in the spinal cord. Therefore, a chronic problem in an internal organ may trigger an ache or "referred pain" in a corresponding area of the back.

Exercise: Prolonged, strenuous or unaccustomed exercise can strain the back muscles. This strain can lead to soreness and tightness.

Improper Lifting: By improperly lifting an object, you can easily strain, twist, or even pull your back out of alignment. Many problems occur when people bend over from the waist and use only their back muscles to lift an object as they straighten to a standing position. It is important to bend your knees as you reach for the object and to keep your back straight as you return to an upright position. This allows the muscles of your legs to do most of the lifting and avoids straining the back.

Sudden Forces: A significant number of back problems arise from sudden forces applied to a flexed, bent-over spine. This can occur with apparently simple forces such as coughing or sneezing while reaching for or lifting heavy objects. If the force is great enough, a disc could rupture and exert pressure on the nerves where they exit the spinal column. A large ruptured disc is one cause of sciatica, a condition where pain radiates down the buttock and leg, and can be accompanied by numbness, tingling, and muscle weakness on the affected side.

Clothing: Restrictive clothing and high heels can contribute to many back problems. Any clothing that restricts or inhibits you from moving freely should be avoided. For example, rigid leather belts can contribute to back problems. If you wear one regularly and have a back problem, experiment with wearing a cloth or an elastic belt for a month. Further, *make sure that your shoes are low heeled*, comfortable, and cushion your step.

Weather: Many people are not aware of the effects that weather has on their bodies. Cold weather, in particular, can aggravate a back problem since the muscles tend to constrict. Drafts and dampness can also be detrimental to a bad back. Be sure to keep yourself warm and dry during cold weather.

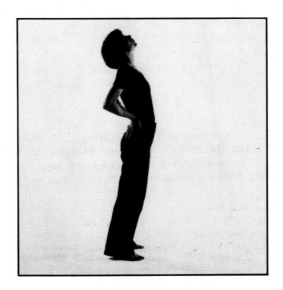

BASIC EXERCISE PRINCIPLES

FOR IMPROVING THE CONDITION OF YOUR BACK

- Make your movements slow, graceful and rhythmic. Be aware of your body and your posture.

- Keep a calm and alert presence of mind. Allow yourself to let go of your other involvements and responsibilities while you practice these exercises consciously. The therapeutic benefits increase when your mind and body work together.

- The spine must be stretched in all of its six possible directions: bending forward, backward, to each side, and twisting to each side. This creates a balance and symmetry in the spinal column.

- When you do an exercise that stretches the spine in any one direction, be sure to follow it with one that stretches it equally in the opposite direction. Beyond this principle, practice these exercises in any order you like. There is no particular sequence to follow.

- Choose to practice the exercises that you enjoy. Do the ones that suit your physical condition and style. Be sure not to overdo any one particular exercise. Gradually work up your physical condition to develop stamina.

- If you exercise longer than a few minutes, allow yourself to completely relax on your back with your eyes closed for a few minutes at the end. You may want to comfortably bend your knees, placing your feet on the floor. Deep relaxation serves to enhance the benefits.

- The exercises themselves can be practiced at various times of the day, easily fitting into your daily schedule. This is a great advantage, because you don't have to practice them at a regimented time.

Constant daily practice is the way to a healthy, flexible back. Start slowly and enjoy the movements. After one month of doing these exercises every day, they will become part of your daily routine, something you'd miss if you didn't do them. The results you experience will motivate you to continue.

Back Care Measures

Posture:

Good posture involves an elongation of the spine. To accomplish this, imagine that a straight cord is being pulled directly upwards from the top of your head. Tilt your pelvis slightly forward and allow your shoulders to relax. Check your posture from time to time throughout the day, making sure your spine is straight and your body relaxed.

Alignment:

Spinal alignment is necessary for a healthy back. When the spine is "out," major muscle groups must compensate and nerves may be pinched. If you think that your spine is out of alignment, see a holistic chiropractor or osteopath for an adjustment. Deeply relax on your back afterwards. Practice the self-help exercises in this booklet to stabilize the adjustment. An awareness of your posture and an effort to improve it is also important for maintaining proper alignment.

Exercise:

The body is designed to move. Problems occur when it doesn't get used. Movement naturally lubricates the spinal column. Stretch and get some exercise every day.

Sleep:

Since approximately one-third of our time is spent asleep, it is an important consideration for back care. Sleep on a flat, firm, comfortable mattress. It is best to use little or no pillow. Do a couple minutes of hip rotations and various stretches before getting into bed. This will help adjust and relax your body for the hours to come.

Shoes:

Wear comfortable, supportive, low-heeled shoes with good arches. The soles should be thick enough to cushion your feet.

Breaks:

Whether you work, study or watch television it is important to take breaks and allow yourself to move and stretch. This helps to relieve stiffness, tension, and improves the general circulation.

Section I

Self-Help

Guidelines for Designing a Self-Treatment Plan:
- Choose three or four exercises that relate to your problem, using the index or the chapter headings in this section.
- Practice these exercises for two or three times a day for one week. Gradually increase the time spent in each posture.
- After the exercises, lie on your back with your eyes closed. Cover yourself with a blanket. Take several slow, deep breaths and allow yourself to completely relax for ten minutes.

Acu-Yoga is the most effective form of self-treatment for spinal disorders. These time-tested exercises work the spine in all directions to promote flexibility and strength. In the practice of Acu-Yoga, the spine often adjusts itself naturally as each vertebrae is systematically moved and the spine is stretched. This prevents uneven pressure on the spinal discs, the pads that cushion and separate the individual vertebrae. Immobility and inflexibility of the spine, along with poor posture, result in spinal misalignments, degeneration of the discs, and pinched nerves. By practicing Acu-Yoga, you can improve the condition of your spine, and of your muscles and organs as well. Daily practice promotes longevity and enhances the beauty of the face and body.

A WORD OF CAUTION: Anyone with a back problem should be sure to practice Acu-Yoga carefully, to move slowly and gently into and out of the postures. This is especially important for people who have long-term, chronic back problems, or people who have back injuries caused by an accident. No exercise should be practiced in a jolting or jarring fashion; no exercise should be pushed beyond your limit. STRETCH—DON'T STRAIN! If you are straining, you are doing it wrong! Do an exercise to the extent that it feels good, somewhere in between pain and pleasure. If a stretch "hurts good," then the level is right for you.

For example, say the pose is "to support your lower back and bend backwards." This **does not mean** that to practice the pose "correctly" you should be in an extreme position—it means to gently stretch into the position as far as you can without straining. If the most you can do is bend your knees and tilt your head back, fine! Then that's your pose. ACU-YOGA IS NOT A CONTEST! Let go of your expectations and accept yourself the way you are.

Gradually, slowly **ease into** the postures. Keeping your eyes closed allows you to get in touch with what you're doing, so that you can feel if you need to back off a little, go a little farther into it, or stay where you are for the moment. Appreciate what you **can** do, because if you accept your level and continue practicing, you automatically become more stretched out, more flexible. Accept, love and appreciate what you are, and you will naturally improve problems in the back.

Tensions in the upper back often have a psychological source. Curvatures, aches, or pressure in between the shoulder blades can be an expression of (1) the internal pressures created by pushing ourselves too hard, or (2) hurtful feelings lodged in back of the heart where the emotions of grief or loss are stored. In the first case, people who continually drive themselves to do more than they can handle are constantly creating internal pressures and tension. What they do is never experienced as "enough." Consequently they have difficulty letting up the pressure on themselves. These inner pressures eventually cause knots of tension in the upper back, mostly between the shoulder blades and in the shoulders.

The second case is of people who do not allow themselves to experience the feeling of loss or grief. Emotionally they tend to hold on to whatever has passed out of their lives. This difficulty in letting go automatically restricts the breath. As emotional holding clamps down on the breathing and the emotional expression of the feeling, tensions around the chest and upper back result.

The Acupressure points in the upper back are related to the heart as well as to the lungs. For example, people with heart conditions or asthma almost always have tension in the upper back. By releasing the tension and balancing the energy, the heart and lungs benefit.

Self-Help for the Upper Back

The upper back is one of the most difficult areas to reach on yourself in order to apply finger pressure. For self care, try placing a tennis ball or a smaller, harder ball such as a racquetball beneath the tender areas as you lay on your back and breathe deeply. You can also ask a friend to *gradually* press directly into any "knots" in your upper back.

These knotted areas are often Acupressure points and may be quite tender at first touch. Maintain a firm but gentle pressure on these points for one to five minutes or until any soreness diminishes and and the "knots" begin to relax and disappear.

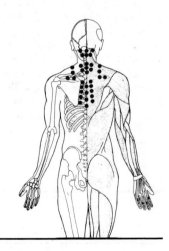

Acupressure points on the hands and arms, held with the upper back points, often help facilitate this release.

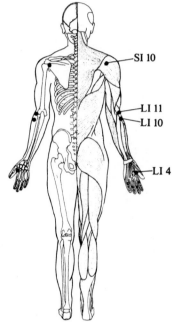

SI 10

LI 11
LI 10

LI 4

SI 10 releases the shoulder girdle and upper back area, traditionally used for hypertension, insomnia, anxiety, nervousness, arm pain or numbness, cold hands.

LI 11 helps to relieve constipation, depression, upper back pain, brachial or intercostal neuralgia.

LI 10 is traditionally used for muscular spasm in the arm or upper back, indigestion, swollen or stiff neck, poor circulation.

LI 4 has been used to relieve neck pain, headaches, migraines, toothaches, constipation, arthritis, neuralgia.

Also practice the following Acu-Yoga exercises. Spend ten minutes twice a day for three weeks practicing these exercises along with utilizing tennis balls to apply pressure between your shoulder blades. Allow two minutes for each exercise and three minutes with the tennis balls. Then spend about five minutes relaxing your back and breathing deeply into your chest.

Upper Back Opener

Stand with your feet about shoulder width. Inhale as you interlace your fingers together behind you. Exhale as you bend forward and raise your arms up behind you. Stretch your arms upward, moving your shoulder blades toward one another. Inhale as you lower your arms and return to a straight standing position. Continue the exercise several times.

Benefits:

This is an excellent exercise for hypertension, upper back and shoulder tension, cold hands, arm problems, anxiety, and insomnia.

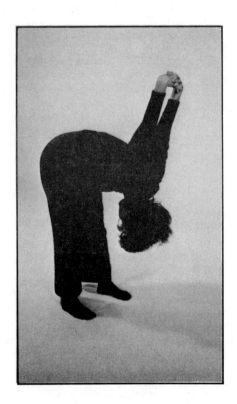

Pelvic Raise

Lie on your back with your legs bent and your feet flat on the floor. Inhale and raise your pelvis upwards. Exhale and slowly come down. Repeat the exercise several times.

Benefits:

This Acu-Yoga exercise not only benefits the spine and many of the inner organs, it also effectively releases muscular tension in the shoulders.

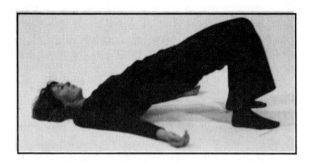

Shoulder Blade Press

1. Sit on your heels.

2. Lower your forehead slowly to the ground.

3. Interlace your fingers behind the small of the back with the palms facing each other.

4. Inhale and raise the arms upward to a 90 degree angle with the hands clasped.

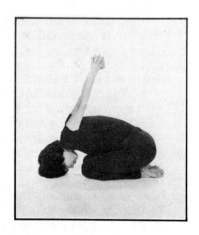

Benefits

This is an excellent exercise for the upper back. Long deep breathing into the chest will therapeutically massage the Acupressure points in between the shoulder blades and on the upper back. After one minute inhale and stretch the arms back. Exhale as you lower the arms down. Relax on your back with your eyes closed for a couple of minutes to discover and assimilate the benefits.

NECK TENSION AND PAIN

The neck is one of the first areas of the body where tension becomes evident. This is part of an ancient reflex from the time when stress arose from physical danger and tensing the neck area helped protect the head and the exposed blood vessels on the throat. Although most stress today is caused by situations that don't require a physical response, the old patterns still function. Thus, whether the stressful situation is primarily physical, mental, or emotional, we still respond by unconsciously tightening the neck muscles.

Further, the feelings that go along with these pressures and demands of everyday life often remain unexpressed, resulting in corresponding emotional tensions. These blocked feelings, and other unfinished emotional business, are also stored in the neck.

Since many people either do not know how to relieve this stress, or don't practice the techniques that they do know, the tensions build and can become chronic. Neck tension, pain, stiffness, and even pinched nerves in the neck are therefore very common. This tension can affect us on all levels, and we become more closed physically, emotionally, mentally, and spiritually. Since the neck is an area prone to accumulation of tension, it is especially important to practice techniques to unblock it.

Self-Help for the Neck

There are many self-help techniques for tight or contracted neck muscles. A combination of (1) Acu-Yoga, (2) hot compresses, (3) deep breathing, and (4) Acupressure have been found to be particularly effective. First apply the hot compresses to your shoulders and neck until the skin becomes reddish. Ginger compresses (see page 103) are highly effective for relaxing the muscles in this area. After applying the hot compresses, rotate your head very slowly five times in one direction and then the other. Keep your eyes closed and breathe deeply as you do this exercise. This will help to elongate the neck and naturally reposition the vertebrae in the cervical region. Next, lie down on your back, placing your hands underneath your neck to press the Acupressure point B 10 (see diagram), located one finger's width outside of the spine on the upper portion of the neck. To find the point, start from the outside of the two large rope muscles that run parallel to the spine and press in very gradually and up towards the base of the skull. If you have severe neck tension, you may also find, in this area, small hard lumps about the size of a pea. Hold the tightest point on your neck for three minutes as you breathe deeply. Then relax with your hands by your sides for another few minutes. For adequate self-treatment, continue this routine for six weeks, practicing two to three times daily. If you suffer from whiplash, be sure to use self-help techniques only after inflammation of the neck has diminished.

Neck Press

1. Lie on your back. Clasp your hands together behind your neck.

2. Exhale, and slowly pull the head up, using your arm muscles. The heels of the palms should be firmly pressing the sides of your neck.

3. Breathe deeply, keeping your head up and your elbows as close together as possible for one minute.

4. Inhale deeply and hold for the count of ten, stretching your neck further.

5. Exhale and slowly lower the head to the floor. Relax with your arms by your sides, eyes closed, and discover the benefits.

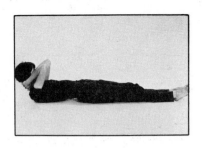

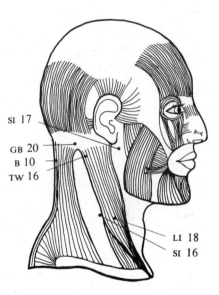

Benefits:
Sore throat, acne, stiff neck, thyroid irregularities, congestion or itching in the throat, mental disorders, speech problems, general pain.

Acu Points	Traditional Associations
Gall Bladder 20	Neck painful or stiff, headaches, insomnia.
Large Intestine 18	Cough, shortness of breath, sore throat, pain in the opposite hip.
Small Intestine 16	Spasm in the neck and shoulder, lethargy, inability to twist the neck due to stiffness.
Small Intestine 17	Swelling and immobility of the neck, sore throat, nausea, tonsillitis.
Triple Warmer 16	Shoulder, back, and arms painful, stiff neck, face swollen, eyes painful.
Bladder 10	Head heavy, spasms in the neck muscles, nose blocked, swollen throat.

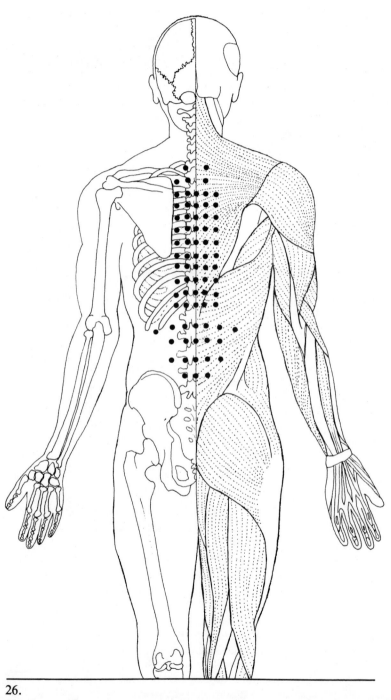

THE MIDDLE OF THE BACK

Emotions commonly associated with the middle of the back include frustration, anger, lethargy, apathy, and worry. Tension caused by an excess of these emotions can adversely affect the digestive and respiratory systems. For example, the spinal nerves in the mid-portion of the back connect to the liver, gall bladder, spleen, and stomach; therefore, any tension in that area will affect these digestive organs. Tension in the middle back can also interfere with the diaphragm and your ability to breathe deeply.

Self-Help Exercises

Exercises and movements that stretch and flex the mid-back not only help to relieve problems in this area and strengthen this portion of the back, but can also increase general vitality. The Acu-Yoga exercises found on pages 30-35 include six which should be practiced once or twice daily to benefit your middle and lower back. Do *Hip Rotations* (page 30) and *Lower Back Bends* (page 31) several times throughout the day. They are done while standing and only take a few minutes. *Cat Cow* (page 33) increases flexibility in the mid-back area. *Flattening the Lower Back* (page 32) elongates while *Dollar Pose* (page 34) actually presses the muscles of the lower and middle back. This helps to relieve tension in those areas. Then finish this series of exercises with *Rock and Roll* (page 35) which massages the entire length of the back.

Acupressure Points

There are three types of Acupressure points which help to relieve pain and tension in the mid-back area; (1) frontal points in the solar plexus area, (2) local points in the mid-back and (3) distal points on the limbs. These three types of points complement each other. In other words, if you press a distal point on your foot before doing an Acu-Yoga posture for the mid-back, the local and distal points work to release one another. The following Acupressure points are beneficial for the mid-back region.*

Lv 3 called "supreme rushing," a distal point for the mid-back, is beneficial for allergies, headaches, insomnia, muscle spasms or cramps, and depression.

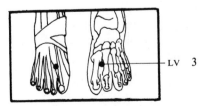

LV   3

---

*An effective strategy for releasing tension in the mid-back is to apply heat to the constricted area. Hot compresses on the back can make Acu-Yoga and Acupressure techniques even more beneficial. Do not apply heat to inflamed areas of your back. Otherwise, hot compresses are generally beneficial for relieving back tensions. (See p. 103.)

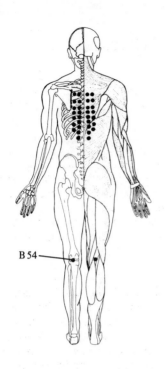

B 54

B 54 called "equilibrium middle" is a key point for relieving mid and lower back pain and tension, especially when pressed in combination with one or more of the local back points illustrated above.

GV 26 called "the middle of man (woman)" is an appetite suppressant point, and helps with hay fever as well as mid-back tension and pain.

GB 24 called "sun-moon" is good for hiccups, snoring, and indigestion as well as tension in the mid-back and diaphragm.

CV 12, 13, 14 associated with the solar plexus, are helpful for easing chronic tension in the mid-back region. Do not press these points on a full stomach.

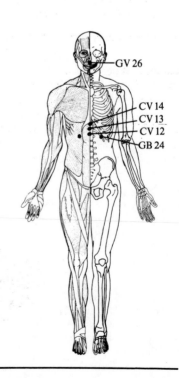

GV 26
CV 14
CV 13
CV 12
GB 24

THE LOWER BACK

Although the majority of lower back problems are directly related to stress, poor posture, accidents or weak musculature in the abdominal region, traditional Chinese medicine teaches that pain or tensions in the lower back are associated with the bladder, the kidneys, and the reproductive system.

The kidneys are considered the storage tanks of the body, gathering surplus energy and storing it to be used when needed. When the kidneys have an abundance of this reserve energy, the lower back will be strong and flexible. However, deficiency or weakness in the kidneys—brought on by "running on nervous energy," eating too much salt, drinking too much liquid or not drinking enough, excessive sexual activity or excessive fear—can cause problems in the lower back area.

Self-Help

The following Acu-Yoga exercises relieve tension and strengthen the lower back. If you have lower back pain, follow the instructions for relieving "severe lower back pain" (page 36) and do Acu-Yoga exercises *Flattening the Lower Back* (page 32) and *Warming the Vitals* (page 31). These exercises are designed to relieve lower back pain. Then gradually work towards practicing the other exercises in this section, which are helpful for lower backaches, stiffness, and tension. Remember to breathe deeply, as instructed.

Sexuality and the Lower Back

In its highest form, sex is an expression of love, tenderness and intimacy. When it is used solely for sexual sensation and gratification, with no sharing and caring, problems and dissatisfaction are inevitable. When people treat each other as sex objects, love making is reduced to a mutual masturbation which sooner or later becomes unfulfilling and, on some level, emotionally stressful. This kind of sexuality fosters anxiety, insecurity, and other negative feelings. The inner pressures of expectations, fears, and lack of confidence tend to accumulate in the lower back region. Love, trust, and intimacy are necessary for a satisfying, long-lasting relationship as well as for a healthy, stable lower back.

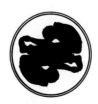

EXERCISES FOR MIDDLE & LOWER BACK

Hip Rotations

Move your hips around in a full circle. Rotate your pelvis several times in one direction and then the other. Breathe deeply and enjoy the movement.

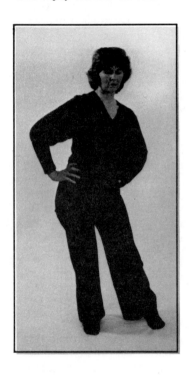

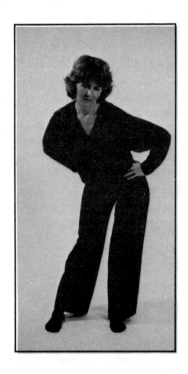

Benefits:

This exercise can prevent many lower back problems. The movement stretches the muscles in the pelvis and lower back. People who have lower back problems with accompanying tension or stiffness should do the exercise several times a day. Make the movements slow and easy without pushing yourself.

NOTE: If you have acute pain from an accident or injury, hip rotations may not be advisable. Consult a physical therapist with any individual questions about these exercises.

Lower Back Bends

Stand with your legs one foot apart with your feet facing straight ahead. Inhale, bringing your hands to your waist with your thumbs pressing your lower back. Exhale as you gently bend back. Inhale again as you straighten up. Exhale as you let the weight of your upper body bring you forward with your head near your knees. Inhale up, exhale down. Repeat the exercise five times.

Benefits:

This movement aids in the flexibility of the spine and benefits the kidneys. It is excellent for fatigue.

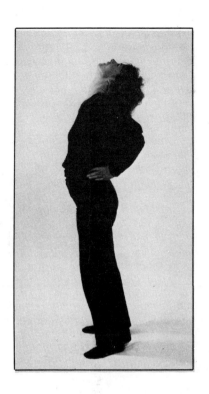

Warming the Vitals

Lie on your back. Place your hands one on top of the other, under the sacrum at the base of the spine. Breathe deeply into your lower abdomen for one minute. Deeply relax with your hands by your side and your eyes closed to discover the benefits.

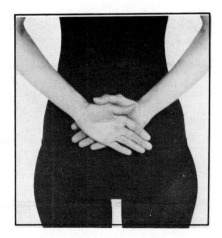

Lower Back Twists

Begin on your back with your legs bent, feet flat on the floor. Exhale as you let your knees fall to the left and your head turns to the right. Inhale as you bring both your knees up to the center. Exhale and let your knees and hips roll to the right. Continue several more times, alternating sides and breathing with the movement.

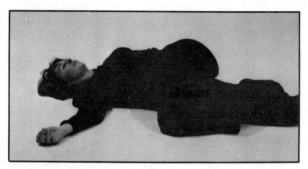

Benefits:
This movement gently stretches the lower back. It also helps to readjust the lumbar spine.

Flattening the Lower Back

Lie on your back with your legs bent and your feet on the floor. Inhale, then exhale, contracting your buttock muscles and pulling in your abdomen so that your lower back presses against the floor. Repeat this several times.

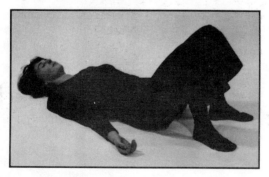

Benefits:
This exercise flattens and elongates your back. It is excellent for preventing lower back aches if there are no problems with protruding vertebrae or degenerating lumbar discs.

Cat Cow

Kneel on all fours. Inhale as the head goes back while you arch your spine. Exhale as the head comes down and the spine curves up. Make the movement rhythmic.

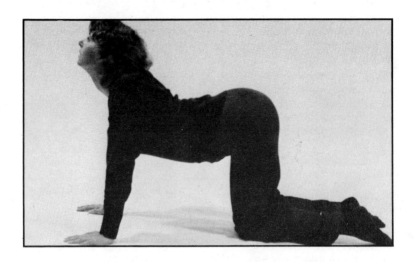

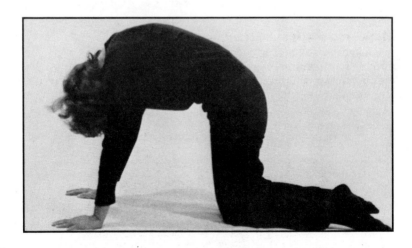

Benefits:

Cat Cow is an exercise that flexes the lower thoracic and lumbar vertebrae, strengthening the lower back and the reproductive organs.

Dollar Pose

1. Lie on your back with your feet together.
2. Inhale and raise your legs up over your head.
3. Use your hands to hold both sides of your heels.
4. Adjust the angle of your legs by bending your knees to apply pressure on the tensest area, either between the shoulder blades or on your mid-back.
5. Relax in the posture and breathe long and deep for one minute.
6. Completely relax on your back with your eyes closed for a few minutes, feeling your blood and energy circulate.

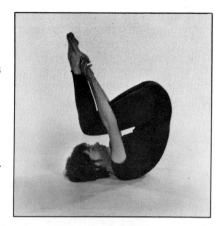

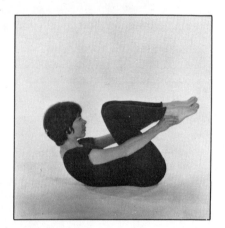

Benefits:
Backaches, stiffness all over, rheumatism, nervousness, anxiety, insomnia.

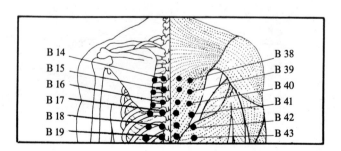

Acu Points	Traditional Associations
Bladder 14-19, 38-43	Hypertension, upper back pain

Rock and Roll

Do this exercise on a padded surface. Bring your arms underneath your thighs and clasp hold of one wrist. Bring your knees to your chest and lean back, tucking your head into the chest. Rock back and forth from the base of the spine to the tops of the shoulders. Use the weight of your legs to propel the body back and forth. Inhale coming up, exhale as you go back.

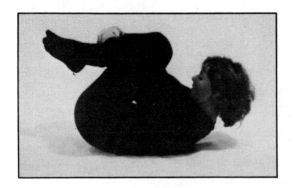

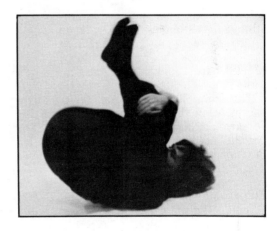

Benefits:

Rocking on the spine this way works on all 94 traditional Acupressure points on the back. Try rocking back and forth for one full minute to relieve overall back tension. Then relax on your back with your eyes closed for a couple of minutes to enhance the benefits of this exercise.

Severe Lower Back Pain

Lie on your back, resting your lower legs on a chair with your knees bent. For maximum relief, you should hold this position for ten to fifteen minutes, breathing slow, deep breaths. Afterwards, lie on your side and bend your knees to your chest until you have completely relaxed for five minutes. Hot pads and compresses (see page 103) are also helpful for relaxing muscular spasms and for improving circulation.

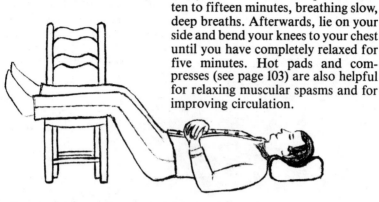

Special Lower Back Pain Point

There is a special point on the arm for relieving aches and pain in the lower back. This point requires strong, firm stimulation. In order to effectively relieve an ache or pain in the lower back this point should be pressed hard enough to be momentarily painful.

This point is located four finger widths below the elbow crease of the forearm. Place all four fingers together (as a measure) with your index finger against the elbow crease. The point will be on the middle of your forearm, just outside your little finger. You will feel a muscular band or cord. The point is directly under this muscle.

To make sure you have the right muscle, wiggle the middle finger of the arm on which you are searching. Press directly onto the muscle that "pops out" and hold firmly for five seconds; it will be momentarily painful. Stimulate this special point on both arms to relieve pain in the lower back.

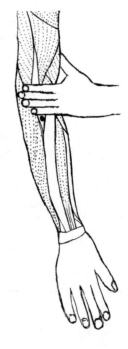

Lower Back Dietary Considerations

There are foods which are detrimental as well as foods which are therapeutic for the lower back. White sugar, for instance, is one of the greatest enemies of the lower back. Metabolizing sugar puts a strain on the adrenal glands, which are located directly on top of the kidneys, with which they are closely linked. Eating or drinking sugary foods like carbonated sodas affects the blood sugar levels adversely and taxes the spleen, pancreas, and kidneys. This puts an additional strain on the lower back.

An excessive or deficient intake of fluids can also tax the lower back area. The kidneys, which control the lower back region, are associated with the water balance in the body. Contrary to Western thinking, too much liquid is detrimental to the kidneys. An excess amount of fluids (especially alcoholic beverages) can overwork the kidneys and weaken the lower back. Therefore, it is best to drink moderate amounts of liquid.

Diet has an important role to play in improving the condition of the lower back. A common Oriental dietary therapy for preventing lower back problems involves preparing beans medicinally; black beans are especially beneficial. The beans should be soaked overnight before cooking and the soak water discarded. The beans should then be cooked in fresh water for an hour and a half. Do not add salt until the last fifteen minutes of cooking time. After cooking beans for about one-half hour, skim off the blackish soot. Eat two to three tablespoons daily for a month, then every other day for the next two months to benefit a lower back problem.

Correct Breathing for Lower Back Problems

The breath is the key to health. Deep breathing exercises are particularly important for developing a strong lower back (see page 97). Breathing deeply increases the amount of fully oxygenated red blood cells.

Many people spend a great deal of their time indoors, both at work and at home, and therefore get very little fresh air and exercise. Even if you live in an area that suffers from air pollution, it is better to get outside at least some time during the day to stretch, move, and breathe deeply.

How you breathe is important for strengthening the condition of your lower back. Tight chest and lower back muscles constrict the ribs so they cannot work properly, causing people to breathe shallowly. When this muscle tension is released, the lungs can open to allow deep, full breathing. This further oxygenates the blood and increases vitality.

Self Acupressure Massage

In a standing position place your fists on both sides of the lower back and gently but briskly rub 100 to 200 times. Continue to rub from your lower back to the buttocks with the backs of your hands until your lower back feels warm. Practice this self Acupressure massage technique two to three times daily.

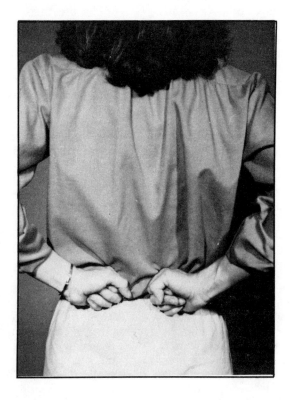

The spine, or vertebral column, is the foundation of the body. It is composed of 33 vertebrae:
- 7 neck (cervical)
- 12 trunk (thoracic)
- 5 lower back (lumbar)
- 5 fused bones at the base of the spine (sacral)
- 4 in the tail (coccyx)

The spine supports the entire body, protects the central nerve cord, and registers the youth and health of a person.

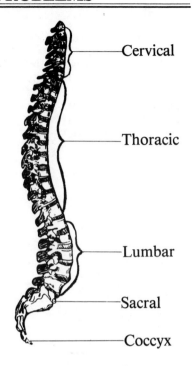

Cervical

Thoracic

Lumbar

Sacral

Coccyx

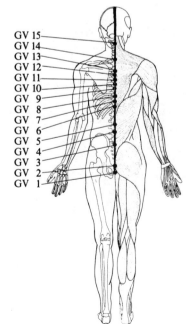

GV 15
GV 14
GV 13
GV 12
GV 11
GV 10
GV 9
GV 8
GV 7
GV 6
GV 5
GV 4
GV 3
GV 2
GV 1

The Governing Vessel: The Master of the Spine

One of the most important Acupressure meridians, the Governing Vessel (GV), runs directly over the spine. This meridian and the spine strongly influence each other's overall strength and balance. Keeping the spine flexible and strong has a direct and positive effect on the Governing Vessel and a beneficial effect on the spinal column and central nerve cord. Similarly, a problem in one can cause a problem in the other. The healthier the spine, the healthier the whole person.

Yu Points

The nerves that go to all parts of our body, and control all the functions of the organs, branch out from the spinal cord, lodged inside the bony vertebral column. There are also the "Yu" Acupressure points that relate to all of the internal organs and functions.

The Yu Points are located close to and on both sides of the spine, between the spine and the large sacro-spinalis muscles that run alongside it.

NOTE: The points are generally located near the associated organ. Each specific area of the back relates to the internal organ that is nearby. Imbalances in the back can affect the organ, and problems in the organ can affect the back. In this way, back problems can express what is happening internally in the body. Pressure on these Yu points can benefit their corresponding organs as well as the spine itself.

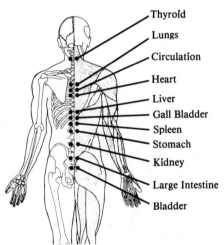

Thyroid
Lungs
Circulation
Heart
Liver
Gall Bladder
Spleen
Stomach
Kidney
Large Intestine
Bladder

The following exercises work on the Governing Vessel, and the "Spinal Flex" especially stimulates the spinal nerve cord which branches out down from the brain. This nerve cord is protected in the bony vertebrae by three layers of membranes and the cerebrospinal fluid that flows between them, which also flows through the brain itself. The "Spinal Flex" exercises flexes and extends the spine back and forth, gently stretching the spinal muscles that hold the vertebrae in place. This enables the cerebrospinal fluid to circulate freely, and improves the condition of the spine and of the back muscles.

Spinal Flex

1. Sit on the heels, placing the top of the right foot over the arch of the left foot.
2. Place the palms on the thighs, with the spine straight.
3. Inhale and flex your spine forward. Arch the spine gently but firmly in this motion.
4. Exhale and let the spine slump back. This stretches the spine in the opposite direction. Let your head simply rest on your neck, moving slightly with each flex of the back.
5. Continue for one minute. Begin slowly and gradually, feeling the motion and stretch in your back. Gradually increase speed as your back loosens up. Breathe with each movement, inhaling as the chest pushes open and forward, and exhaling back and down.
6. Completely relax on your back for a couple of minutes.

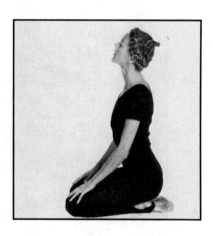

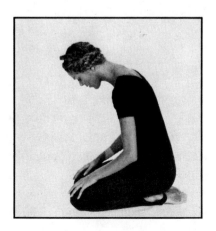

Benefits:
Relieves spinal stiffness, back aches and pains, indigestion, nervous disorders, postural problems, nervousness, and cold feet.

Spinal Twist

Sit straight on a chair or on the floor. Turn your head and upper body to the left. Use your right arm to grasp your left thigh and pull as a lever to get a good twist. Use your left arm to support the body as shown. Repeat the twist for the other side. Breathe out as you twist to the side.

Benefits:

This is a good stretch to do first thing after getting up out of bed in the morning. The spine is most relaxed at this time. This gentle stretch helps to realign the vertebrae in the lower back.

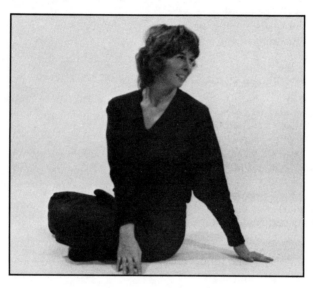

CAUTION: This exercise is not recommended for severe lower back problems such as a ruptured disc. Please consult your osteopathic doctor, chiropractor, or physical therapist.

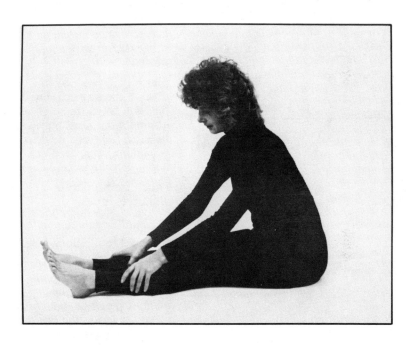

Life Nerve Stretch

Sit with your legs together, stretched out straight in front of you. Keep your knees straight. Exhale and lean forward. Inhale up and exhale down several times. The deeper you breathe, the easier it is to stretch the back and legs.

Lie back and relax for a few minutes. Be sure to follow this exercise with "Cobra Pose" (on page 44) to stretch the spine in the opposite direction.

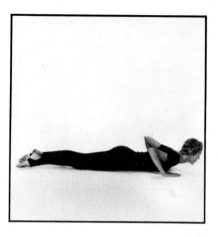

Cobra Pose

1. Lie on your stomach with your feet together and your chin on the floor. Place your palms on the ground underneath your shoulders.

2. Inhale slowly, lifting your head up and stretching the neck. Continue inhaling, and raise the chest, using both the arms and the back muscles.

3. Finish the inhalation and arch all the way up. Your hips will be on the ground, your arms may be either bent or straight, depending upon the flexibility of your spine.

4. Exhale in this position, and begin long deep breathing for about 30 seconds, gently pressing the navel to the floor.

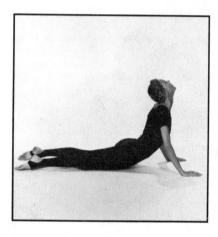

Cobra Pose stretches the spine to increase its flexibility, release tension, and prevent scoliosis. It stimulates the nerves of the back to balance all the internal organs. Cobra Pose is also good for nervousness, headaches, hypertension, impatience, and sexual imbalances.

5. Using your arms for support, lower yourself partway down so that the segment of the spine that needs the most attention receives some pressure. Hold the body at this angle, breathing deeply into the blockage in the spine for another 30 seconds.

6. Slowly come down all the way, letting your head rest on its side, and your arms by your sides. Close your eyes and completely relax for several minutes.

The Acu-Yoga postures work on all the various parts of the spine. The cobra pose, for example, usually works on the lumbar vertebrae of the lower back. A variation on the same pose, however, can be beneficial for the upper back. This traditional posture can affect all segments of the spine, from the sacrum at the base to the topmost vertebra in the neck.

Acu-Points	Traditional Associations	Area that Benefits	Inches from the Ground (Chest to the Floor)
Governing Vessel 15 & 16	Neck stiff, rigid, headache, colds, speech problems, fear, suicidal.	Cervical (neck)	3-5 inches head back
Governing Vessel 11, 12, 13, 14	Nervousness, spine rigid and painful, eyes heavy, neck, shoulders and back painful.	Upper Thoracic (upper back)	6-9 inches arching chest out
Governing Vessel 6, 7, 8, 9, 10	Back pain, lower back especially stiff, limbs weak, hypertension, cardiac pains.	Lower Thoracic (middle back)	10-12 inches ½ way up
Governing Vessel 4 & 5	Lumbar pain, impotence, vaginal discharge, loins and back stiff and painful	Lumbars (lower back)	12-15 inches almost completely up
Governing Vessel 1, 2, 3	Lower back painful, extreme nervousness, irregular periods, lumbago, colitis, abdominal distension.	Sacrum (small of the back)	15-18 inches all the way up & buttocks contracted

Plow Pose

Lie on your back with your legs straight, your feet together. Inhale and raise your legs up at a 90 degree angle from the ground. Reach your arms up to grasp hold of your ankles. Move your legs to the angle that puts pressure on a tense area of your back. Breathe deeply into the tightness. After 30 to 60 seconds come out of the posture slowly by supporting your lower back with your hands. Completely relax on your back for a couple of minutes.

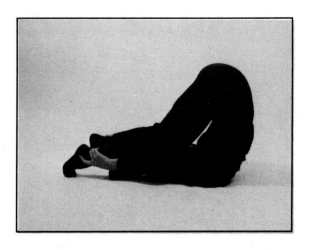

Angle of Pose	Area of Release	Traditional Associations
90 degrees	Mid-back	Liver, gall bladder problems, overeating, aggression, repressed anger and postural problems.
60 degrees	Upper back	Cardiac problems, high blood pressure, insomnia, and self imposed pressures.
45 degrees	Shoulder blades	Resistance to colds and flus, chills, fever, and changes in the weather.
Toes above head. On the floor,	Top of shoulders	Thyroid conditions, neck and shoulder tension, depression or uptightness.

A unique advantage of Acupressure self-care is its accessibility; you can easily apply it in your daily life, no matter what your lifestyle. Acu-Yoga exercises do not have to be practiced strictly in a regimented scheduled way. A lack of space or time or a comfortable rug on the floor does not have to deter you from incorporating these exercises into your life. A few minutes of quiet time is all you need.

Many self-Acupressure techniques can be used spontaneously, whenever you want or need them, at any time. At work, for example, you may discover that there are certain postures or ways of working which actually create tension. Acupressure points and Acu-Yoga stretches are helpful tools for learning new ways of sitting or standing that do not cause tension.

The exercises in this section can be practiced anywhere there is a place to sit, whether in a chair at home or the office, or even while sitting in a parked car. Often just taking a couple of minutes to practice simple exercises like the Neck Press and Elbow Lift will have a dramatic effect on reducing tension and stiffness and at the same time improve your outlook on life.

Upper Back Opener

Sit up straight with your buttocks at the edge of the chair. Bring your arms behind you and interlace your fingers. Inhale, and let your head drop back. Straighten your arms and lift them away from your lower back. Exhale, bring your head forward and relax your arms. Repeat two more times.

Benefits:

Uptightness, upper back and shoulder tensions, insomnia, difficult breathing. This exercise also strengthens resistance to illness.

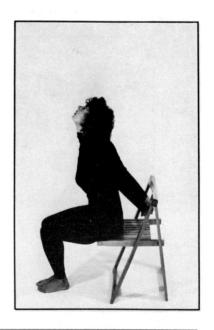

NOTE: You will find some of these exercises in other sections of the book, shown in a standing up or lying down position. All of the exercises can be adapted in this way.

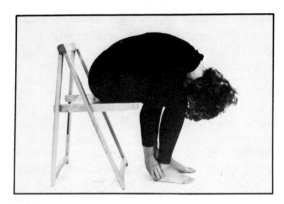

Dollar Pose

Gradually bend forward. Grasp both sides of your heels. Lower your head toward your kneecaps, fitting them into the eyesockets. Take three to five deep breaths in this position.

Benefits:

Lower and mid-back pain or stiffness, eye strain, appetite imbalance and general fatigue.

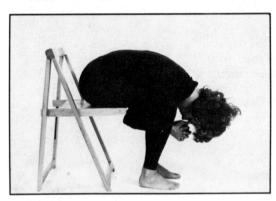

Back Curl

Bend forward bringing your arms underneath your knees. Drop your head forward, allowing your neck to relax. Use your thumbs to press underneath the eyebrows at the bridge of the nose. Continue to hold this point as you take three to five deep breaths.

Benefits:

Sinus headaches, overall back tension, overeating, fatigue, and constipation.

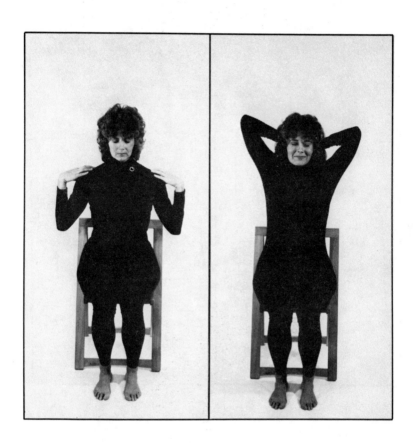

Elbow Lift

Place your hands on your shoulders. Right hand on right shoulder, left hand on left shoulder, with your elbows out to the side. Inhale and lift your elbows straight up and towards each other. Exhale as you relax down. Repeat three times.

Benefits:

Shoulder and neck tension, fatigue, irritability, and cold hands.

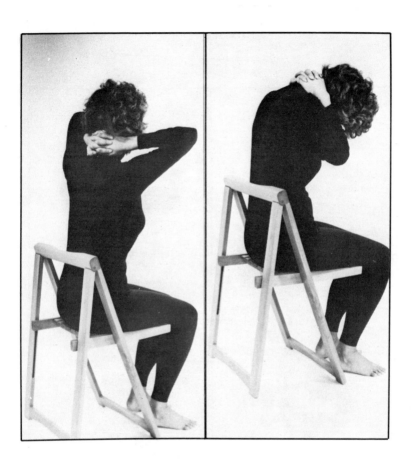

Neck Press

Interlace your fingers behind your neck. Slump downward and bring your elbows in towards each other. Inhale as you raise your elbows upwards. Exhale and slump downward again. Take three long deep breaths with the movement.

Benefits:

Chronic neck tension, insomnia, headaches, repressed anger, irritability, nervousness, acne, and sore throat.

Spinal Twist

Inhale and cross your legs at your ankles or your knees. Exhale and twist to one side, grasping the back of the chair with one hand, the outside of the knee with your other hand. Inhale as you face forward. Exhale twisting to the other side. Repeat once more in each direction.

Benefits:

Pressure or stiffness in the lower back, colitis, constipation, and abdominal distension.

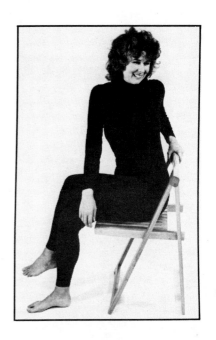

Ankle Press

Squeeze the achilles tendon from the base of the calf to the ankle, twice on each side. Finish by rotating your feet five times in both directions.

Benefits:

This stimulates distal points on the ankle beneficial for relieving back tension, swollen ankles, cold feet, and urinary-reproductive difficulties.

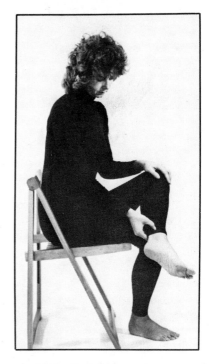

Section II

Back Points
for Specific Conditions

NOTE: Although this section is organized symptomatically, it contains valuable information that can apply to everyone, not just to those who have the particular symptom.

What to Do After a Back Injury

Immediately after an injury, ice is often applied to the area to reduce pain and swelling. Hot compresses can be used to relieve pain accompanied by stiffness or muscular contractions but should not be used when there is inflammation.

It is most important not to strain yourself further after a back injury. The healing process naturally takes time. Care for yourself with plenty of rest and proper nutrition; then gradually increase the time and intensity of the Bum Back exercises to rebuild the strength and flexibility of the spine.

Acupressure helps to relieve the muscular contractions that accompany a back injury. If a portion of the back is particularly sensitive, use only light touch in that area. Do not press directly on open wounds, bruises or inflamed areas. As the back becomes stronger, deeper pressure on the points will be appropriate. Points not located on the back can also be helpful for emotional trauma that often follows a back injury. Hold each of the following for approximately three minutes while breathing slowly and deeply.

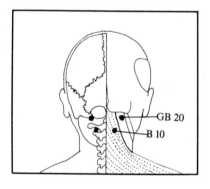

GB 20, called the *Gates of Consciousness*, is located just below the base of the skull, in a hollow between two muscles. This first-aid point is often used after injuries to relieve pain and trauma. It is a key point for headaches, back pain, insomnia, nervousness, mental pressures, and neck tension.

B 10, called *Heavenly Pillar*, is located on the upper portion of the neck, approximately one thumb's width outside the spine. Usually a lump of tension can be felt at this point. It is a key point for releasing stiffness, rigidity, and pain in the neck and back. This Acupressure point also strongly benefits the nervous system and is especially useful in times of stress and trauma.

Points for Trauma & Back Injuries

CV 17, called the *Sea of Tranquility*, is located in the center of the breastbone (sternum) in a hollow at the level of the heart. This point relieves anxiety, nervousness, hysteria, and trauma. Light to firm contact at this point is calming, soothing and relaxing.

CV 6, called the *Sea of Energy*, is located between the navel and the pubic bone on the mid-line. Gradual, deep pressure (to about one inch) at this point strengthens the general condition of the body. Acupressure on CV 6 can accelerate recovery from a back injury.

P 6, called the *Inner Gate*, is located two finger widths above the center of the inner wrist creases. This point is helpful for balancing the emotions and the internal organs. It has traditionally been used for nausea, appetite imbalances, indigestion, emotional trauma, dizziness and insomnia.

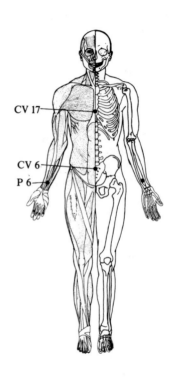

Complementary to Acupressure is Reflexology, deep breathing, visualization, and meditation.* Pressure on the Reflexology points stimulates the nerve endings in the feet, hands, and ears. This triggers a healing response in the injured area. Long, deep breathing oxygenates the blood, improves circulation, reduces pain, and internally massages the back muscles. Practice the deep breathing, visualizations and meditations in this book and get plenty of rest to maximize the healing process after a back injury. You cannot force recuperation, but you *can* encourage it by paying attention to the needs of your body.

*Reflexology: see pp. 100-102.
Deep Breathing and Visualization: see pp. 97-98.
Meditation: see pp. 99.

Special Back Release Points

Like the Governing Vessel which connects the Acupressure points along the spine, the Bladder Meridian governs the back muscles. It connects points from the head down through the neck, back, back of the legs, and the feet. Acu-

pressure on any Bladder Meridian point can benefit a back problem. Therefore, the areas behind the thighs, the backs of the knees and in the center of the calves contain points for the back. Prolonged finger pressure (three to five minutes) on these points allows tension and pain to drain from the back. Use the points illustrated to help relieve back pain regardless of where it is located.

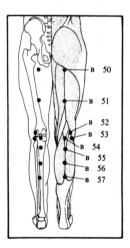

Also, use these points to complement the release of back tension with either Acu-Yoga or Shiatsu. Gently stretching the backs of the legs as well as holding these points can help alleviate back tension, stiffness, aches and pains.

Acu Points	Traditional Associations
Bladder 50	Hemorrhoids, constipation, lumbago, sciatica, pain in the back.
Bladder 51	Inability to bend up and down easily, pain in the back and loins.
Bladder 52, 53	Muscular spasm of the calf, knee and loin pains.
Bladder 54, 55	Body feels stiff and heavy, stiff back and neck, arthritis of the knee.
Bladder 56, 57	Pain in calf and instep of foot, muscular cramps.

Benefits: sciatica, urinary and bladder problems, stiffness or pain behind the knee, muscular spasms, cold feet, late afternoon fatigue, leg stiffness or pain.

SCIATICA

Sciatica refers to a pain which runs down the back of the leg, beginning in the hip or buttock(s) region and traveling down the back of the thigh or along the side of the leg. This pain may extend below the knee and reach as far as the ankle or foot. Pain from sciatica can be intense enough to immobilize someone. Walking or bending in certain directions can be painful. Some people experience numbness in certain areas or pain in the lower back. Sciatic pain can be caused or aggravated by a lack of mobility in the pelvic region, lower back strain, excess frustration, injury to the lower back, causing a lumbar disc to protrude or a misalignment of the sacroiliac joint or lower lumbar region.

Acupressure along with gentle manipulations has proved to be effective for relieving as well as preventing sciatica. Pelvic movements which gently stretch the buttocks muscles and lower back area complement the tremendous therapeutics of Acupressure for relieving sciatic pain.

Self-Help Techniques for Sciatica

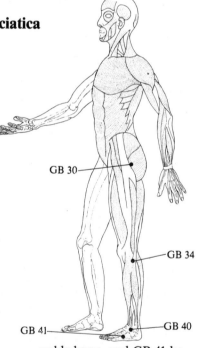

Lie on your back and place both fists underneath your lower back so that the knuckles are pressing into the lower back muscles. Hold for one minute. Then roll over onto your side, placing your fist or a tennis ball underneath the side of your buttocks. This point (GB 30) is one of the key points for relieving sciatica. The pressure on this point should create a pain that "hurts good." Close your eyes and breathe deeply for several minutes. Readjust the pressure as the soreness decreases, pressing other tight points in the area. This should be followed by pressing three points: GB 34 (a muscle relaxant point) located on the outside of the lower leg below and in front of the head of the fibula, GB 40 in the indentation directly in front of the outer ankle bone, and GB 41 between the fourth and fifth metatarsals, just below the juncture where the bones begin to narrow on the top of the foot.

The following Acu-Yoga exercises help to prevent sciatica. They should be practiced twice daily for best results. These exercises are also beneficial for people who already have sciatica and back pain. If you have sciatica, practice the following exercises* slowly and with awareness; don't push yourself beyond your limits. Be sure to utilize long, deep breathing:

- **Hip Rotations,** page 30
- **Lower Back Twists,** page 32
- **Spinal Twists,** page 42

• **Leg Swing:** Stand next to a chair. Place your left hand on the back of the chair. Shift all of your weight onto your left foot and swing your right leg backwards and forwards. Swing your leg freely like a pendulum. Make sure that you do not swing your leg to the side, as this will strain your back. After about thirty seconds, switch sides and swing the other leg. The purpose of this exercise is to promote greater circulation and mobility in the hip joint.

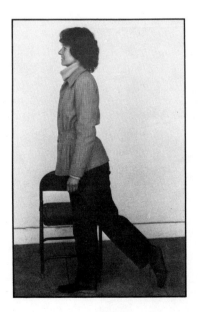
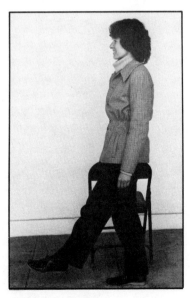

---

*IMPORTANT: After practicing these techniques, allow yourself five to ten minutes of deep relaxation, lying on your back with your eyes closed. Remember, relaxation enhances the benefits.

Helping Someone with Sciatica:

Have the recipient lie on his or her back. Kneel close to the outside of the recipient's right thigh. Use your left hand to pick the leg up from underneath the knee as you support the recipient's foot with your right hand. Gradually bring the recipient's knee towards his or her chin. Instruct the recipient to breathe long and deep as you rotate the knee in a slow circular motion, first in one direction and then the other. Begin with small movements about one foot in diameter, then gradually increase the size of the circle. The intent is to stretch the tendons and muscles in the pelvic region and promote circulation in the sacroiliac joint. Finish the movement by *slowly* bringing the right knee over to the left side of the recipient to twist and stretch the lower back. Do not make any fast or jarring movements. Slowly stretch the muscles in the hips and lower back, then lower the right leg to the ground. Repeat the rotation on the left aside, allowing three to five minutes per side. These rotations, along with the use of Acupressure on the hips and pelvis, are some of the most effective forms of alleviating sciatica, especially if it is chronic.

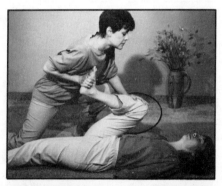

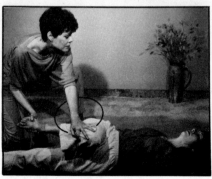

Shoulder and Neck Tension

Many of the Acupressure meridians travel through the neck and shoulder region. This is often the first area of the body where tension accumulates when someone is under stress.* Anyone with

pressures, such as deadlines, obligations and taxing responsibilities, usually suffers from shoulder and neck tension to some degree. A "pain in the neck" is often the body's literal response to these frustrating situations.

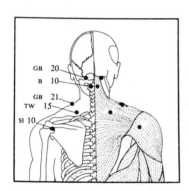

GB 20
B 10
GB 21
TW 15
SI 10

The release of shoulder and neck points improves circulation and is especially good for cold hands, fatigue, irritability, shoulder pains and stiffness of the neck. Traditionally, these points are also considered useful for hypertension.

Acu Points	Traditional Associations
Triple Warmer 15	Shoulder and neck pain, arm and elbow painful and cannot be raised, stiff neck.
Gall Bladder 20	Alternately hot and cold, eyes foggy, nervousness, painful shoulder, rheumatism, stiff neck, upper parts of the body feel heavy or hot.
Gall Bladder 21	The major point where shoulder tension collects. Traditionally used to release stiff neck, regulate hyperthyroidism, and relieve rheumatism.
Bladder 10	Head heavy, spasm of the neck muscles, limbs and body not coordinated, throat sore or swollen.
Small Intestine 10	Muscular pain, numbness, swelling or arthritis in the shoulder—scapula region.

*Refer to page 24 for more information on neck pain.

Cardio-Vascular Problems

Emotional stress is often stored in the upper back, particularly on the large ropy paraspinal muscles between the shoulder blades. Chronic tension in the upper back can eventually constrict or weaken the heart and be a contributing factor in hyperten-

sion. The following Acupressure points benefit not only the cardio-vascular system in general, increasing circulation into the arms and hands, but they also aid in reducing anxiety, difficult breathing and insomnia.

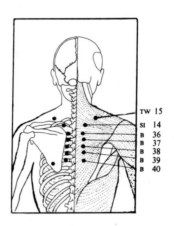

TW	15
SI	14
B	36
B	37
B	38
B	39
B	40

Acu Points	Traditional Associations
Bladder 36, 37	Shoulder spasm or pain, bronchitis, brachial neuralgia, lungs weak, weary and paralyzed.
Bladder 38, 39, 40	Asthma, all types of cardiac disease, slight fever, spasms in the upper back.
Small Intestine 14	Muscular pain and neuralgia of the shoulder and arm, a sensation of coldness circling the shoulder, pneumonia.
Triple Warmer 15	Chest troubled and melancholic, shoulder and back painful, arm and elbow pain when moved.

Digestive Difficulties

Along the midsection of the back at the level of the lowest rib, there are Acupressure points on the Bladder meridian that strongly influence digestive problems, helping to relieve indigestion, stomachaches and abdominal bloating. These points along with other Bladder points on the lower back aid the urinary and reproductive systems as well. When we become fa-

tigued or exhausted, tension accumulates in the lower back. Exercising and stretching these areas with Acu-Yoga can not only relieve this back tension but also increase your general level of vitality.

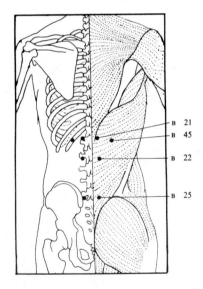

Acu Points	Traditional Associations
Bladder 45	Abdomen distended.
Bladder 21	Stomachache, indigestion.
Bladder 22	Bowels congealed, abdominal pain.
Bladder 25	Constipation, intestinal gas.

Benefits: lower back pain, ache, or stiffness; sciatica, fatigue, urinary disorders, groaning, belching, snoring, complaining, constipation, poor digestion, overeating.

Sexual–Reproductive Problems

Nerves connect many of the Acupressure points at the base of the spine with the sexual and reproductive organs. Firm, prolonged pressure on these points will ease muscular tension in the pelvis and increase the circulation of blood to the genitals and the lower limbs.

These points help relieve menstrual cramps, labor pains, hip pains, sciatica, sexual impotency and urinary and bladder disorders.

Deep frustrations often get stored in this area. Stimulation of the points around the sacrum also aid in the secretion of sex-related hormones for strengthening the sexual and reproductive organs in both men and women. When these points are released a sense of well-being pervades.

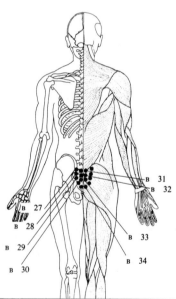

Acu Points	Traditional Associations
Bladder 27	Disorders of the sacroiliac joint, colitis.
Bladder 28	Retention of urine, pain in lumbosacral area.
Bladder 29	Kidneys weak, back stiff, impotency.
Bladder 30	Lumbago, sacral pain, sciatica.
Bladder 31, 32, 33, 34	Constipation, lumbago, impotency, sterility, vaginal discharge, genital diseases.

Benefits: constipation, lower back disorders, pain or pressure at the base of the spine, abdominal weakness, sciatica, bladder and sexual reproductive weaknesses.

Acupressure During Pregnancy

Using Acupressure points can effectively relieve lower back aches and pains as well as other discomforts that can occur throughout pregnancy and labor. The most important areas to emphasize are the buttocks and lower back. Points in these areas should be held from three to five minutes with firm, prolonged finger pressure. Women who are pregnant can either hold these points on themselves or ask somebody to help. For self-help refer to page 106 to design your own back roller for pressing these back points.

Points for Pregnancy

The points illustrated below are helpful for relief of morning sickness, insomnia, back aches, abdominal discomfort and labor pains.

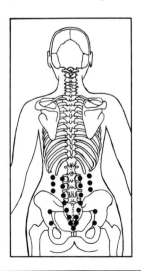

Forbidden Points

Several Acupressure points should not be stimulated during pregnancy. Although the following points may be touched or lightly massaged, it is advisable not to strongly rub or press them during pregnancy: Sp 6, Sp 9, Cv 12, LI 4, St 36, GB 21.

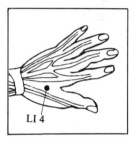

LI 4

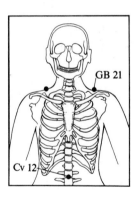

GB 21

Cv 12

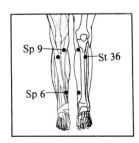

Sp 9

St 36

Sp 6

Acupressure Points for Relieving Menstrual Tension

Many women experience lower back aches and abdominal tension just before or during menstruation. Holding the following Acupressure points often helps to relieve these symptoms.

Sp 12 and 13: Two very important points for releasing any symptoms of menstrual discomfort are located in the pelvic area. These points, which are next to each other, are found in the groin one finger width directly above and one finger width below the crease formed when the leg is bent. Use your finger tips to feel for tension in the area, about one hand width from the midline. Sp 12 and 13 are often very tender when any kind of menstrual tension exists. A few minutes of finger pressure on these points combined with deep breathing is particularly effective for cramps and abdominal discomfort.

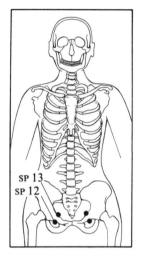

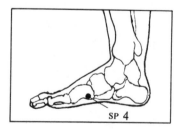

Sp 4: This Acupressure point, traditionally used for menstrual tension, also corresponds to the foot Reflexology area that relates to the back.

It is located on the arch of the foot about halfway between the big toe knuckle (first metatarsal-phalanges joint) and the front of the inner ankle bone. Feel for a protrusion at this halfway point and press around it until you find the sensitive spot. Several minutes of firm pressure on this point can be helpful for menstrual and abdominal cramps, intestinal swelling and stomach aches. This point is also used for foot cramps and cold feet.

CV 1: Located in the center of the perineum, CV 1 has traditionally been used for both vaginal and perineal disorders. These include pain in the vagina, prolapse of the vagina, dysmenorrhea (pain with menstruation), amenorrhea (lack of menstruation) as well as irregular menstrual periods. Pressure on this point not only helps to relieve general tension in the lower abdominal area, but can also release pain at the base of the spine.

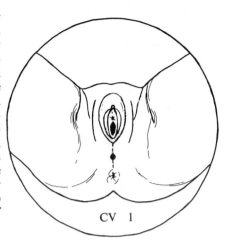

CV 1

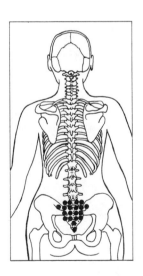

Sacral Points: The Acupressure points on the sacrum are also helpful for relieving menstrual cramps and lower back pain. The points are located in the tiny holes of the sacrum, the broad triangular bony structure below the small of the back. These points are directly related to the reproductive system, via the sacral nerves. Steady, firm pressure on the sacral points can help to relax the uterus and relieve menstrual cramps.

Shiatsu for Menstrual Tension

The Shiatsu techniques in the Acupressure For Others section, pages 71 to 80 can easily be adapted for menstrual tension by simply concentrating the massage on the lower back and buttocks.

Acu-Yoga Self-Help Techniques

Practice of Acu-Yoga strengthens and releases tensions in the lower back and buttocks and can thus help to prevent and reduce menstrual discomfort.

"A moderate regimen of regular exercise that strengthens the back and abdominal muscles can dramatically reduce menstrual back ache within a few months"[1]

Barbara Seaman and Gideon Seaman, M.D.

Constant practice of Acu-Yoga over a period of time can also stimulate the endocrine system to regulate the hormones associated with menstrual difficulties.[2]

For Preventing Menstrual Cramps		For Relieving Menstrual Cramps	
Pelvic Raise	page 23	Severe Lower Back Pain	page 36
Lower Back Twists	page 32	Flattening the Lower Back	page 32
Cobra Pose	page 44		
Cat-Cow	page 33	Breath & Back Roller	page 106
Hip Rotations	page 30	Warming the Vitals	page 31
Lower Back Bend	page 31	Ginger Compresses (for lower or back)	page 103

Dietary Considerations

Calcium is one of the most important minerals for preventing menstrual cramps and for relieving associated lower back pain. This mineral enables the nerves and muscles to relax. Calcium levels drop substantially during the week before menstruation; this low level of calcium can cause pre-menstrual tension, bloating, lower back pain, nervousness, and headaches. Foods that supply the body with calcium can help prevent cramps if eaten during the ten days preceding menstruation. These include fresh green leafy vegetables such as spinach, kale, parsley (which can also be steeped for tea), collards, and turnip greens as well as sesame seeds and tofu (a high protein food made from soy beans).

Magnesium is also important, since it aids in the absorption of calcium. As with calcium, magnesium levels drop during the week before menstruation. At this time, many women experience a craving for chocolate, which contains magnesium. (Chocolate also contains oxalic acid, which blocks the absorption of calcium.) This craving can be eased by including dairy products, sea vegetables (available at health food stores), and a moderate amount of seeds and nuts in the diet. These all contain high amounts of both magnesium and calcium.

1. Barbara Seaman and Gideon Seaman, M.D., *Women and the Crisis in Sex Hormones,* Bantam Books, p. 180. This book contains an excellent discussion of preventive methods for menstrual tension.

2. Please refer to *Acu-Yoga* by Michael Reed Gach, Japan Publications (distributed by Harper & Row), pp. 193-196, for more information on the physical and emotional conditions that can cause menstrual tension.

Section III

Treatment for Others

NOTE: Chronic back problems may need to be worked on every two or three days for the first two weeks. Choose the Jin Shin Acupressure style if back pain is involved. Shiatsu and the Acupressure Massage Techniques are most effective for relieving back tension and stiffness.

TREATMENT FOR OTHERS
USING SHIATSU TECHNIQUES*

There is a great difference in the amount of pressure each person needs. If a person's body has a solid, firm build then use deep, firm pressure. This type of body enjoys deeper pressure. On the other hand, if a person's body is soft or frail then lighter, more sensitive pressure will be appropriate.

Although the right amount of pressure varies from person to person, Acupressure feels exquisite when applied correctly. Many of the Acupressure points lie deep within the body. Press in deeply but slowly. Remember that you are penetrating human tissue that responds to sensitivity and care.

With the recipient in a sitting position:

1. Massage, grasp, knead, and press the shoulder and upper back muscles.

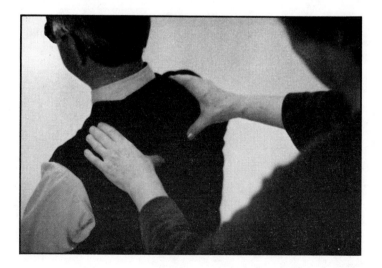

---

*Shiatsu is a Japanese form of massage therapy using pressure on Acupuncture points.

---

2. Glide the palm of your hand down the spine so that your third finger touches each vertebrae. Feel for tensions along the spinal column as the palm goes down the back. This will give you a whole picture of a person's posture and back tensions.

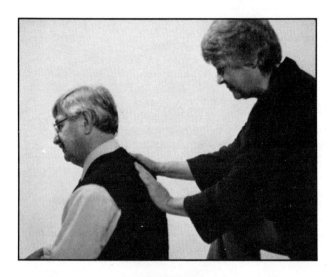

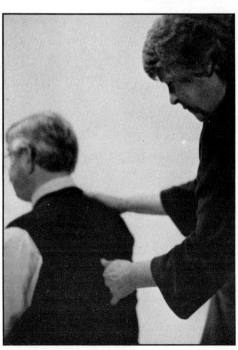

3. Hold the tightest spot with your hand. Support the shoulder with your other hand. Have the person rotate their head around. Hold with steady firm pressure for a minute or until the muscle begins to soften. Repeat exercise #1 and #2 working on another tense area.

4. Elbow Slide

Rest your elbows on the tops of the recipient's shoulders. Glide your elbows ever so slowly down the muscles that run an inch from and parallel to the spine. Repeat the elbow slide three times as the recipient slowly lowers their forehead toward the ground. If the elbows have a tendency to slip down and off the tightest back muscles, you are pressing too hard. By easing up, you will be able to slide down the back with greater control.

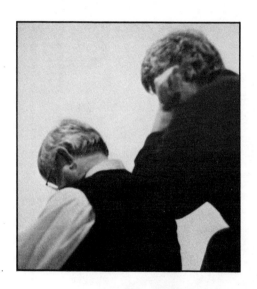

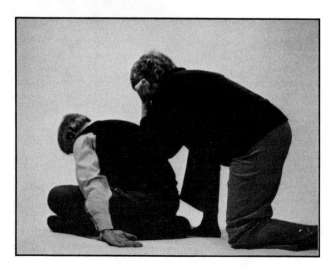

5. Recipient leans forward. Use the heel of your hands with the fingers pointed inward to press the large rope muscles in the lower back and the sides of the buttocks. When you come to a tense spot, ease up on the pressure and move more slowly through the area.

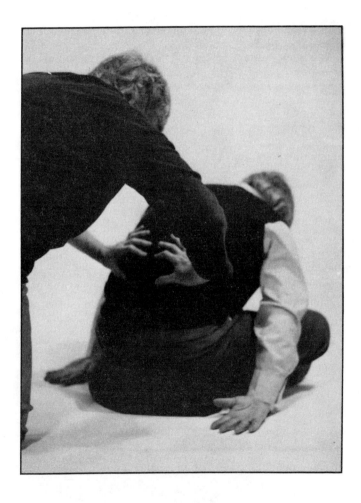

With recipient lying on stomach:

6. Leaning Palms

Place the palms with fingers pointing outward on the upper portion of the back on either side of the spine. Use your body weight to lean into the back with the elbows locked straight. Encourage the person to exhale each time you lean into the back. Establish a rhythm as you gradually move down the spine to the lower back, leaning in with your palms on the exhalation, easing up on the inhalation. This is a most natural technique for overall back tension.

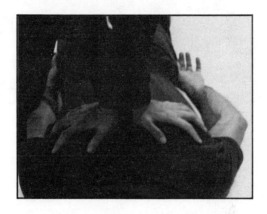

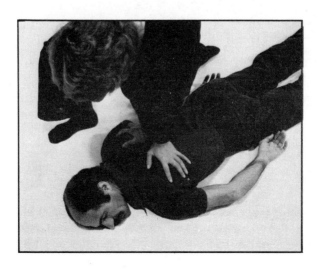

7. Melting the Block

Place the palm of your hand on the tightest part of the back. Maintain firm pressure as your other hand rhythmically presses the buttocks muscles and continues down the leg. Concentrate on melting the tension in the back with the hand that is stationary.

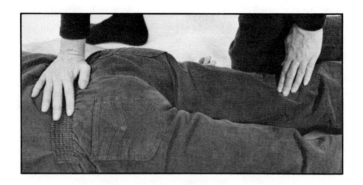

Special Acupressure Point

The point in back of the knee is good for releasing back tensions. Simply hold this point with the fingers of one hand while holding the back with the other hand. Use this special point with the above Shiatsu technique for "melting the block."

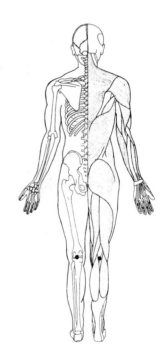

8. Cat Walk

Use the heel of your palms to walk on the back like a cat. Lean the weight of your body into different back tensions. Just let your weight lean into the person. If you weigh less than the person you are working on, then lean more. But if you weigh more than they, lean less. Adapt the pressure according to each individual and area of the body. The most effective pressure is in between pain and pleasure. Gradually apply deep pressure using sensitivity at the same time. This amount of pressure unblocks the tension and stimulates the body to heal itself.

9. Thumbs

Starting at the top of the shoulder blade, place both thumbs along one side of the spine about one inch apart. Move down an inch lower, each time you press in, covering the entire spine.

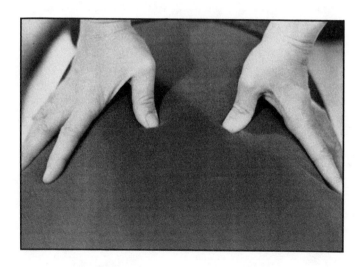

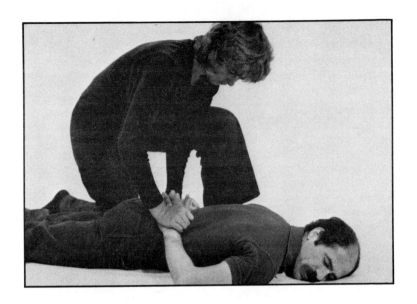

10. Lower Back Massage

Have the recipient lie on his/her stomach. Straddle the body or kneel to one side. Bend over and firmly grasp the recipient's wrists. Use the backs of the recipient's hands to press and massage the buttocks muscles as illustrated. Work up as far as the lower back. Also use the back of your fists to press the muscles in the buttocks and lower back.

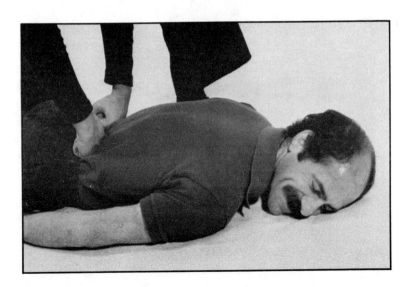

11. Vertebral Push

Sit at the left side. Place the right hand on the center of the back, with fingers parallel to and on the spinal column. Place the palm of the left hand over your right hand so that the hands form a cross. Lean into the body with your palms as the recipient breathes out. Work down the back to the base of the spine, pressing directly on the sacrum.

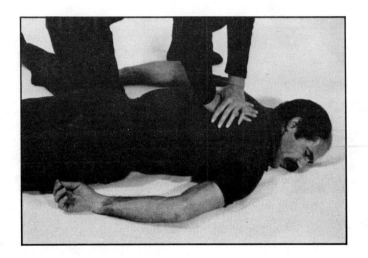

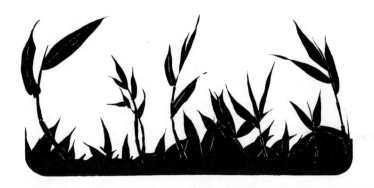

Cradling the Head

Have the recipient turn over onto the back. Sit at the top of the head to finish. Bring the hair out from under the neck. Sensitively knead the muscles at the back of the neck, using your thumb and fingers to squeeze out the tension. This Acupressure massage technique is most effective when done very slowly.

Hold the head in your palms. Let the back of your hands rest on the ground. Support the whole skull with your fingers curved, gradually pulling it outward. Slowly rake the skull, gliding your fingertips over the head. Imagine that the contact of your hands is communication of love and support that words could never say.

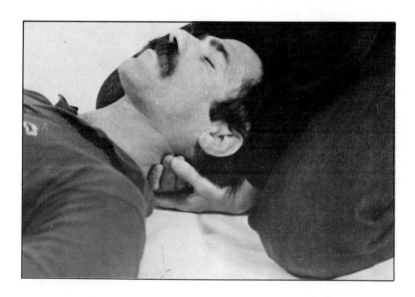

JIN SHIN ACUPRESSURE
FOR THE BACK

Jin Shin, meaning "the art of the compassionate spirit," is a form of Acupressure developed in Japan. It is highly effective for relieving back pain, pressures, and stiffness. Jin Shin stimulates the same Acupressure points as in Shiatsu and Acu-Yoga, but uses fewer points and holds these points for a longer period of time. Usually two points are held at the same time and finger pressure is maintained from thirty seconds to five minutes. Holding two points at the same time is usually more effective than simply holding one since one point helps to release the other. Tension that accumulates around the points is released and circulation to the back is improved.

As you practice the following Jin Shin releases for the back, take your time, breathe deeply, be aware of your own body, and that of your recipient. Hold the points until the muscles in the area soften or until a pulse can be felt. This usually takes a few minutes. Be sensitive to how the recipient feels; ease up if any pain is felt. The amount of pressure will vary from person to person; it should feel good to the recipient, a balance between pain and pleasure.

General Back Release

1. Start with the recipient sitting comfortably. Feel the rope-like muscles which lie along both sides of the spine. Use your finger tips to detect any tense areas in the back and ask the recipient where he or she feels tension, stiffness or pain.

2. Next, have the recipient lie on a comfortable mattress on his or her back with eyes closed. Sit at the side of the person where you felt the most muscle tension or where he or she feels the most pain.

3. Slip your hand underneath the recipient's back to hold the tightest point with your fingers. This point, which is referred to as the *base point*, is held the longest time (for three to five minutes).

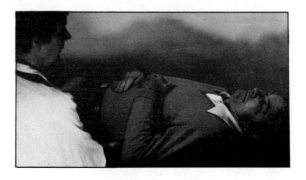

4. Use your other hand to hold the sequence of points illustrated while you continue to hold the base point. (The larger dots on the illustration are the most frequently used points.) All these points (B 36 through B 49) are located on these rope-like muscles described above. When finding a point, simply contact the outside of the muscle cord and gradually press it in and towards the spine. Hold several of these points on the same side of the recipient.

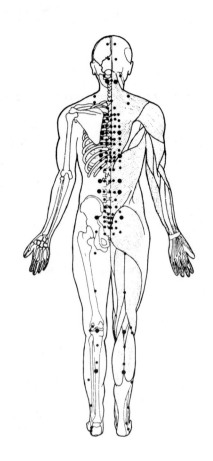

5. Next, sit at the recipient's head and, with your finger tips reach under the neck, on both sides. You will find two muscle bands, one on each side of the spine. With the backs of your hands on the floor, straighten your fingers to press directly up and onto these muscles with your finger tips. Hold the muscles for two minutes. This helps to relieve neck tension and enhances the release of the back.

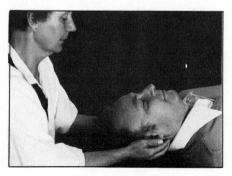

Lower Back Release

1. Have the recipient lie on a comfortable mattress on his or her back, with the eyes closed. Sit at hip level, on the opposite side of the pain or pressure.

2. Place the hand that is closest to the recipient's head underneath his or her lower back. Slide your palm under the spine.

3. There are two rope-like muscles that run parallel to the spine. Curve your hand so that while the heel of your hand presses the muscular cord nearest you, your finger tips contact the muscles on the opposite side. Gradually, very gradually, increase the pressure with your fingers to firmly uplift and press into this muscle.

4. Continue to hold the lower back and use your other hand to hold the following sequence of points (illustrated). Hold each point for at least one minute. Encourage the recipient to breathe deeply into the lower back as you hold these points.

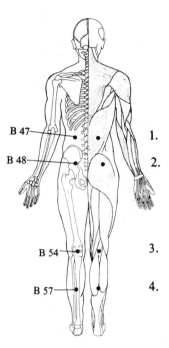

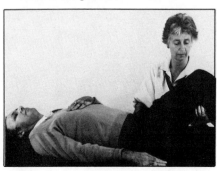

- **B 47** midway between the iliac crest and base of the lower rib, three fingers' width outside of the second lumbar vertebra.
- **B 48** two fingers' width outside of the widest portion of the sacrum.

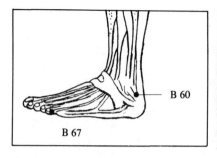

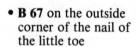

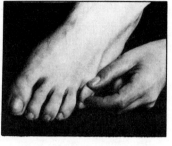

- **B 60** between the outer ankle bone and the back of the ankle

- **B 67** on the outside corner of the nail of the little toe

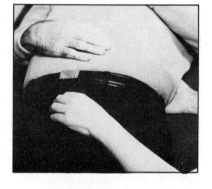

- **CV 6** approximately one inch deep between the navel and the pubic bone, on the midline of the body

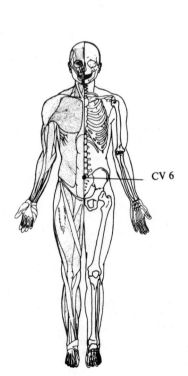

5. Finish with the *master back point* (K 27) located on the upper chest in the small indentations directly below the head of the collar bone. Hold both sides together for one minute. Encourage the recipient to breathe deeply as you hold these points.

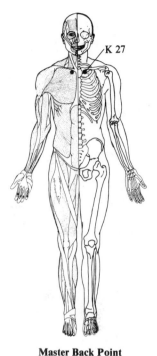

Master Back Point

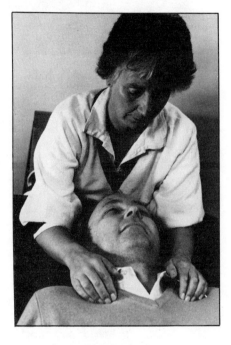

6. At the end of the Acupressure session, cover the recipient with a blanket. Let him or her relax deeply for at least ten minutes. This enhances the effects of the release.

ACUPRESSURE MASSAGE
FOR THE LOWER BACK

Have the recipient lie down on his or her stomach with the head turned to the side, hands by the sides of the body, and a pillow beneath the waist. Encourage the person to breathe deeply to encourage the back muscles to relax.

1. Use the flat of your hand to slowly rub the back, beginning at the pain-free areas and working gradually towards the sore region. Work lightly. Do not cause any pain; only give comfort.

2. Knead the back muscles again, beginning at the pain-free areas, working towards the lower back. Gradually increase the depth of the massage. The amount of pressure to be applied will vary from person to person. It is best simply to ask the recipient for feedback.

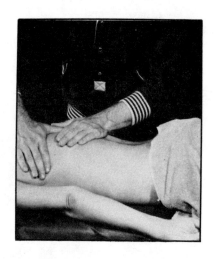

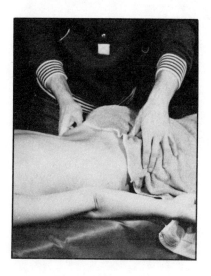

3. Tightness in the buttocks often reinforces lower back problems. So thoroughly knead the buttocks muscles. Next, massage the tension in the small of the back. Spend several minutes manipulating the muscles in this region, using the Shiatsu techniques illustrated on pages 71 to 80.

4. Use your thumbs or fingertips to hold the Acupressure points illustrated. Begin with the points in the lower back (B 23, 47), the buttocks (B 48), and behind the knee (B 54) on both sides simultaneously, holding each for one minute or until the muscle relaxes.

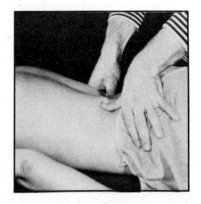

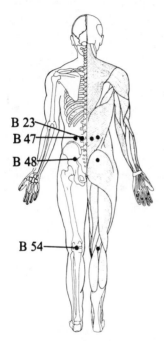

B 23
B 47
B 48

B 54

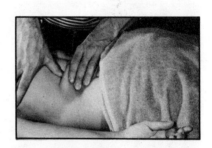

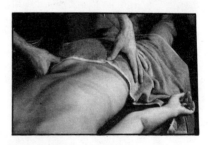

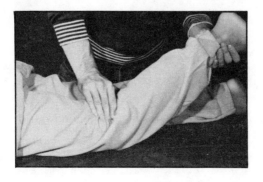

5. Lift both feet up, bending the legs. Slowly press the heels toward the buttocks. Hold the legs in this position for a few seconds, then release by placing the feet down on the ground again. Finish by massaging the ankles and arches of both feet.

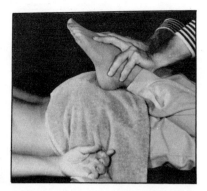

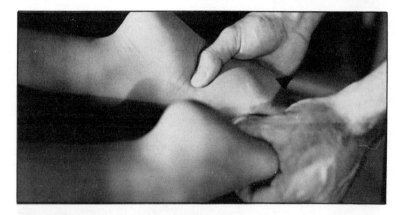

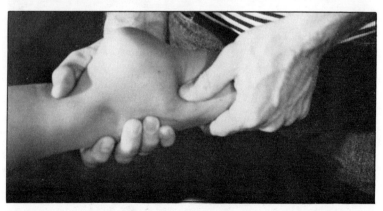

NOTE: If there is severe tenderness in the lower back region, massage the distal lower back points in the legs and ankles. These key Acupressure back points are illustrated on pages 83-84. Gently massage the lower back when the pain and soreness diminish. Acupressure should not be given for lower back aches when there are broken bones, TB of the spine, a slipped disc or bone diseases.

FOR COUPLES

Sitting Back to Back

Sit back to back on the floor with your legs crossed. Close your eyes. Adjust your position so that you can comfortably lean on your partner for mutual support.

Interlock your arms at the elbows. Slowly rock backward and forward with your partner. This exercise can be done with your legs straight out in front, bent at the knees, or cross legged.

Benefits: This exercises stretches the thoracic vertebrae. It benefits the spleen, liver, and gall bladder.

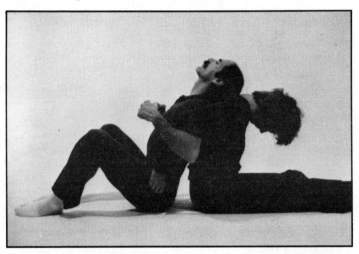

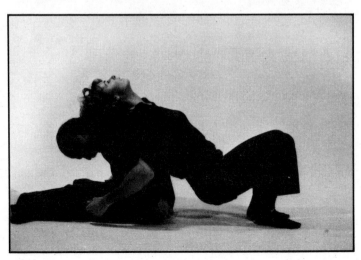

Standing Back to Back

Stand back to back interlocking your arms at the elbows. One person squats a little to get lower and gradually leans forward. The other person leans backward, arching the back. After several seconds both people return to an upright position. Then alternate positions and repeat the stretch in the opposite direction.

Some people will comfortably be able to lift their partner off the ground. It is important to do this exercise slowly without straining.

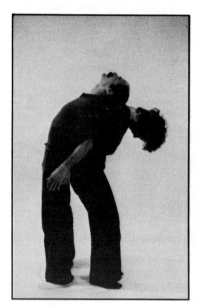

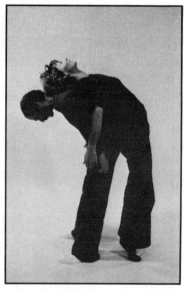

Benefits:

The lower back is stretched and elongated in this partner exercise. It can relieve pressure and pain in the lower and mid portions of the back. The stretch also opens up the chest region.

Lower Back Press

1. Have the recipient lie on his/her back.

2. Bend their legs, pressing the knees together and toward the chest for one minute.

3. Instruct the recipient to breathe slow and very deeply while you are leaning on them in this position.

4. Extend the recipient's legs straight out in front of them. Allow the person to lie on their back with their eyes closed to relax for a couple minutes.

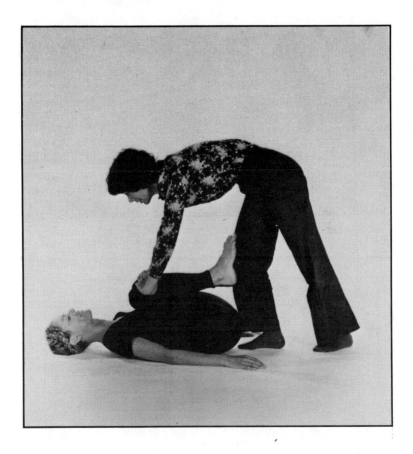

Benefits:

Lower back aches, abdominal distension, constipation, gas, urinary and reproductive problems.

GIVING & RECEIVING

Acupressure not only feels good and is beneficial but brings people closer together. The mutual exchange as well as the release of tensions can be excellent for marital problems and a great way to enhance friendships.

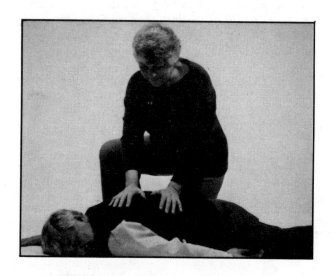

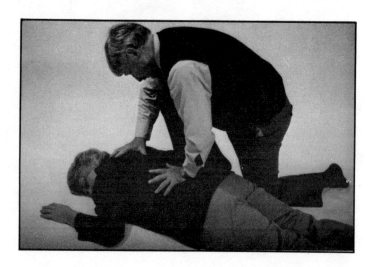

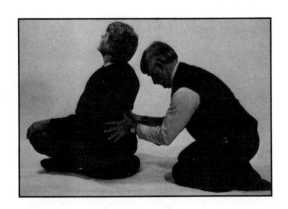

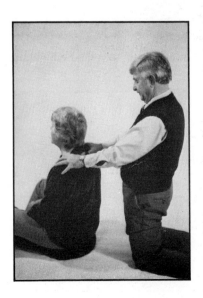

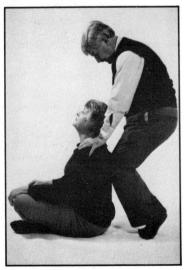

Section IV

Back Care Alternatives:
Methods, Tools & Resources

BREATHING TECHNIQUES

The breath is an important indicator of the way we feel. Since the breathing mechanism is an automatic process, we unfortunately tend to ignore this potent source of life energy and assume that it is operating properly. Naturally, we manage to breathe enough to sustain life, but a greater awareness of our breathing process would lead directly to increased vitality and optimal functioning.

If your posture is poor, your breathing may be shallow and therefore your body's vital systems will be functioning at a diminished level. If you improve your posture and deepen your breathing, your respiratory system can function fully to properly oxygenate the cells of your body.

Further, the breath is one of the most profound tools for revitalizing the back. The following breathing meditations help to reduce your back pain and tension. These techniques can increase your overall effectiveness in life as well. You can do them anytime, even when occupied with your daily activities. Place your attention on your breath and feel the benefits it provides.

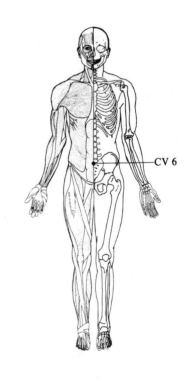

Deep Breathing is the most basic technique for dealing with back pain. Deep breathing balances the nerve and meridian pathways that travel through your back. Inhale deeply into your abdomen, diaphragm, and finally your chest. Hold the breath for a few seconds, then exhale slowly. Consciously breathe slowly, gradually, and deeply, concentrating on making each breath full and complete.

Hara Breathing nourishes the internal organs. It is beneficial for strengthening the lower back and for preventing problems in this area. The *Hara*, known also as the "the sea of energy," is located three fingers width below the navel, at the Acupressure point Conception Vessel 6 (CV 6). Concentrate on this area while breathing deeply into your abdomen. You can lay your palms over the hara to make sure that the lower abdomen rises as you inhale and falls as you exhale.

CV 6

Breath Visualizations help you to use the tremendous power of your imagination to focus on your spine. This can loosen your back and promote awareness, positive attitudes, and greater circulation.

The possibilities are endless. Create a visualization which will benefit your back; you can utilize a combination of color, sound, body parts, guided awareness, and positive affirmations as you breathe. For instance, if you have back pain, picture a sky blue color and imagine bringing that blue color in, with your breath, to the painful area; blue tends to soothe pain. The following are examples of other simple breath visualizations for your back:

Using the Breath to Ease Back Pain

Lie down on your back with your knees bent or sit in a comfortable chair. Close your eyes, and focus on an area of your back that needs attention. Imagine the breath as a substance penetrating that area of your back or spine. Concentrate on breathing into the blockage. If an ache or pain is in your lower back, for example, breathe deeply into those tight muscles. As you inhale, imagine the warmth of your breath relieving your back pain or tension. Hold the breath a couple of seconds at the top of the inhalation. Exhale smoothly, allowing the pain to leave with your outgoing breath. Do this for several minutes, concentrating on making your breath as long and as deep as possible.

The Flute Breathing Meditation

Lie down comfortably on your back with your knees bent or sit in a comfortable chair. Imagine you are breathing into your spine. See your spinal column as a large flute. Concentrate on breathing into this instrument. Make each breath long and deep. Breathe out any tensions you feel restricting your lungs. Feel your back relax as you breathe into your spine.

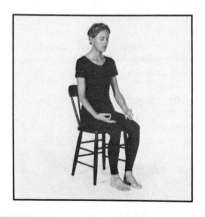

MEDITATION TECHNIQUES

The tranquility achieved during meditation has extensive therapeutic benefits for chronic back problems and other stress disorders. Meditation uses a variety of techniques such as deep breathing, postures, visualizations, and sounds which affect the brain, the nervous system, and in turn, the endocrine glands. This regulates the body's metabolic rate and provides a deep state of internal rest. Over a period of time this can rejuvenate the entire back as well as the central nervous system.

"...In the back are located all the nerve fibers that mediate movement. If the movement of the spinal nerve is brought to a stand still, the ego, with its restlessness, disappears as it were. When a man (or a woman) has thus become calm, he (she) may turn to the outside world. He (she) no longer only sees the struggle and tumult of individual beings, and therefore has that true peace of mind which is needed for understanding the great laws of the universe and for acting in harmony with them. Whoever acts from these deep levels makes no mistakes."*

Concentration is meant to be effortless during meditation. Keep your spine straight and focus consciously on breathing deeply. Allow your inhalation and exhalation to be smooth and complete. Do not ponder the thoughts that come to you. Instead, observe their flow, watching them come into your mind and letting them go. When you notice that you have stayed with any one thought, let it go and bring your awareness back to slow, deep breathing. This continual process of letting go increases circulation to the brain.

Meditation for Strengthening the Spine

The following meditation utilizes the breath and an internal "lock," or contraction, for strengthening the spine.

1. Sit comfortably with your spine straight and your eyes closed.

2. Lengthen your neck by lifting your chest and pressing the chin lightly towards the hollow of your throat.

3. Connect the tips of your thumb and index finger of each hand and rest the backs of your hands on your knees.

4. Inhale deeply. Exhale and at the end of each exhalation squeeze your buttocks for a few seconds, contracting your rectum and pelvic muscles.

5. Continue the deep breathing with the contraction for two minutes.

6. Then simply meditate on your spine as you breathe deeply into your belly.

7. Continue for two more minutes. Be sure to keep your spine straight throughout the meditation.

*Richard Wilhelm, *I Ching* rendered into English by Carrie Baynes, Princeton, New Jersey; Princeton University Press, 1968, page 201.

REFLEXOLOGY
FOR THE BACK & SPINE

Reflexology is a beneficial self-treatment technique that is complementary to Acupressure. The points, similar to those used in Acupressure, correspond to nerve endings and are located on the soles of the feet, the palms of the hands, and on the ears. As in Acupressure, the points in Reflexology relate to and benefit specific areas and organ systems of the body; Acupressure points relate to body parts by means of the meridians while nerve reflex points do so by means of nerve pathways. For instance, when there is an imbalance or weakness in an area of the back, there will be a related area of sensitivity in the corresponding area of the foot, hand or ear. This soreness is often caused by crystallized calcium and acid deposits which accumulate over the nerve endings.

Gradual pressure on these points breaks up and dissolves the crystals. This pressure should feel good but should be firm enough to stimulate the point. This also stimulates the nerves to energize the affected area of the body. The amount of pressure used will vary from person to person and from point to point. For instance, people who eat a lot of processed foods and who do not get enough exercise may have tender spots on their hands, feet, and ears. If so, gradual, prolonged light pressure is best: touch rather than press these points. As the point is held, the tension or crystallized calcium deposit will begin to dissolve and more pressure will become appropriate.

Suggestions for Practicing Reflexology

- Keep your fingernails cut short or work with a dull instrument such as an avocado pit or the eraser end of a pencil.
- When possible, close your eyes in order to relax more, and to really feel the points.
- Avoid distractions. Adjust the light so it is not too bright and make sure you are warm and comfortable.
- Listen to your body. Be sensitive to both the areas which are the most tender and those which need greater pressure.
- The reflex points lie underneath the skin. Note that the size of the points varies, with some covering an area the size of a kidney bean and others no bigger than the head of a pin. Develop your sensitivity to the points through attentive practice.
- Five minutes of deep massage on each foot is sufficient for a person's first Reflexology session. If you work longer than this, too many toxins can be released at once. Be moderate at first to allow the body time to adjust, rebalance and heal.
- Concentrate on what you are doing! Keep your attention focused on the here and now.

Foot Reflexology

Foot massage is especially good for elderly, sick or disabled people with back pain or tension. It feels good to almost everyone, relaxing and rejuvenating the entire body. It helps the circulation so that toxic materials can be released, thus benefiting the blood, organs, glands and nerves.

By massaging and pressing points on the arch of the foot, you can benefit the spine. Use the chart below as a reference when you find a tender spot on the arch of the foot. This spot will often correspond to a problem area in your back. The problem area can benefit by holding the tender spot on the foot until the soreness diminishes.

Also, an excellent natural way to massage the reflex points on the feet is to walk barefoot as much as possible. Walking on grass, sand, earth or smooth rocks naturally stimulates these points. If the soles of your feet are especially tender, it is best to walk barefoot on grass or soft earth, gradually increasing the times until your feet are stronger.

Ear Reflexology

If you have a back problem, you will find a very sore point in your ear that corresponds to that area of your back (see chart below). The right ear corresponds to the right side of the back; the left ear corresponds to the left side of the back. If the pain or problem is in the center or on the spine, then both ears are used. Hold the tender spot for several minutes until the pain diminishes and the spot pulsates or feels warm.

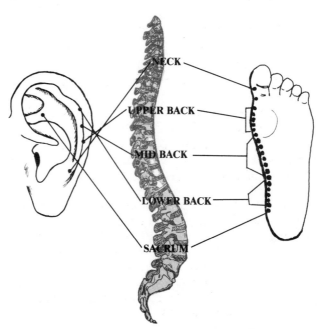

NECK

UPPER BACK

MID BACK

LOWER BACK

SACRUM

Acupressure & Reflexology Hand Points

The hand Reflexology points for the back and neck are located along the index finger and the thumb. The base of the index finger near the wrist corresponds to the lower back or lumbar region. If you have lower back pain, you may find a tender spot in the webbing between the thumb and index finger or in the base of the thumb.

Once you find a sensitive or painful spot in the hand, use steady finger pressure for 2-3 minutes. As you hold the point you may discover that the tenderness disappears. Mildred Carter in *Hand Reflexology* claims: "Relief almost always follows the first treatment, apparently regardless of the cause of the back trouble."*

Use the hand charts below to locate the Acupressure and Reflexology points that relate to your back. Try holding some of the more sensitive points for several minutes until you feel a steady pulse at the point. The pulse may feel faint at first, but continue to hold the point until the pulse becomes strong and balanced. A regular pulse indicates that the point is released, increasing the circulation to heal the corresponding areas of the body.

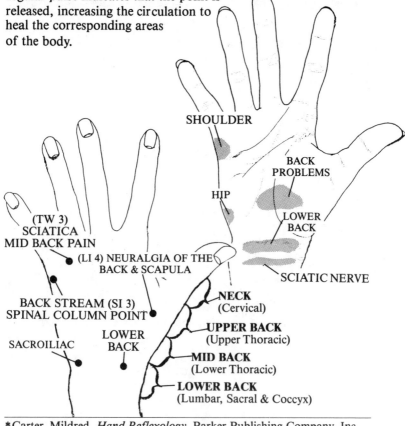

SHOULDER

BACK PROBLEMS

HIP

LOWER BACK

(TW 3) SCIATICA MID BACK PAIN

(LI 4) NEURALGIA OF THE BACK & SCAPULA

SCIATIC NERVE

BACK STREAM (SI 3) SPINAL COLUMN POINT

NECK (Cervical)

SACROILIAC

LOWER BACK

UPPER BACK (Upper Thoracic)

MID BACK (Lower Thoracic)

LOWER BACK (Lumbar, Sacral & Coccyx)

*Carter, Mildred. *Hand Reflexology*, Parker Publishing Company, Inc. 1978, p. 113.

GINGER COMPRESSES
FOR RELIEVING BACK TENSIONS

Fresh ginger is an excellent pain reliever. Ginger compresses are especially effective for releasing chronic muscular tensions in the back.

Heat two quarts of water. Grate a half pound of fresh ginger and place it in a thin cloth that is approximately one foot square. Tie the opposite corners securely and place in the hot water. Make sure that the water does not boil. Let the bag of ginger sit in the hot water for a half hour. Then squeeze the bag to get the juices out of the ginger.

Dip a towel in that hot water. Ring out some of the liquid and gently place it on your back tension. The water temperature should be as hot as you can tolerate without burning the skin. Redip the towel when it cools. Continue to apply the hot packs until the skin becomes reddish pink.

Apply ginger compresses regularly as needed. Long term chronic ailments such as asthma, arthritis, and bursitis may need more applications but can be helped quite easily. Apply the ginger compresses in the upper back for asthma. Apply compresses directly on the tense area of the back. The redness indicates increased circulation.

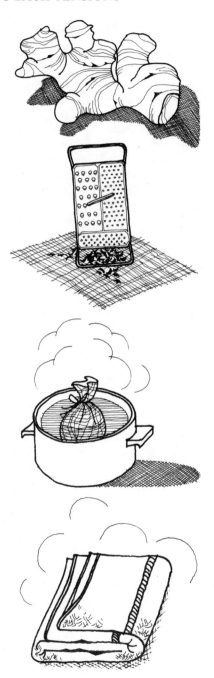

Using Heat to Relieve Back Pain

Often back pains are the most severe in the morning, upon waking. The pain usually eases as the movement of daily activities stretches out the muscles a little. Heating pads or hot baths are helpful in that they provide some temporary relief from pain and stiffness, but they do not usually change the condition more than that, unless used in conjunction with other therapeutics such as Acupressure or Acupuncture. Heat, in combination with regular practice of Acu-Yoga, Shiatsu, and deep relaxation can give both short and long term results. Pressing the Acupressure points with warm towels can loosen up the muscles so that you can get more benefit from the postures. Deep relaxation after practicing Acu-Yoga or Shiatsu balances and stabilizes the body's energies, providing a deep state of rest to enable the back to heal and strengthen.

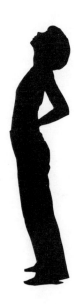

TOOLS FOR RELIEVING BACK TENSION

(Available through the Acupressure Workshop in Berkeley, California)

Ma Roller: A hard wooden roller designed to stimulate Acupressure points along the spine, by lying down on it. Good for someone who likes lots of deep pressure.

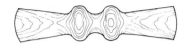

Captain Carrot Caresser: Similar to a rolling pin, with two thick strips of hard rubber padding. Good for "rolling out" your muscular tensions.

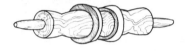

Body Buddy: This small wooden roller has a convenient handle. The Body Buddy is preferred by those who need less pressure for relieving back tension.

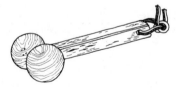

Rubber Balls: Buy a tennis or small rubber ball (about 4″ in diameter) in a dime, toy, or sports store. Simply lie on the ball to relieve back tensions.

CUSTOM BACK ROLLER

Materials:

- One inch thick round wooden dowel or rubber tube, about 12 inches in length

- One large, thick towel

- Two pieces of heavy string or ribbon (2 feet each)

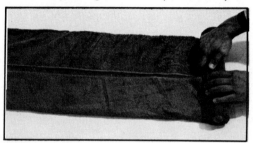

Instructions:

1. Lay the towel out flat. Fold the outer edges in toward the center as shown below.
2. Place the dowel or tube at one end of the towel. Roll the towel up around the dowel.
3. Tie the string around the towel to hold it in place.
4. Place your roller on the ground. Lie down on your back with the roller underneath you.
5. Roll it to an area of your back that feels tense or sore.
6. Stay on that area for about a minute with your eyes closed, breathing deeply and slowly.
7. Move the roller to other tense areas of your back and repeat #6.

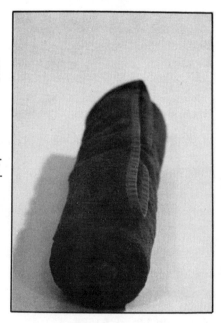

NOTE: Try using tennis balls instead of the tube. Place the balls about three inches apart and roll the towel up around the two balls. Use as directed above.

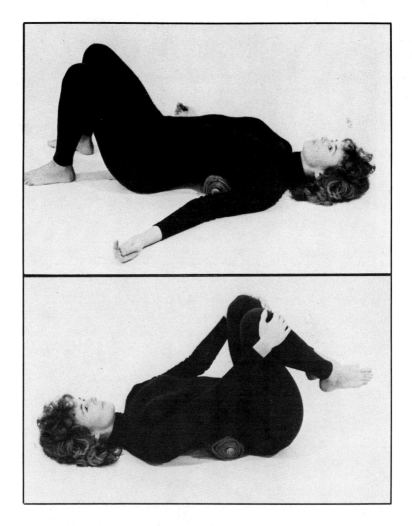

Bringing your knees towards your abdomen will increase the pressure of the roller on your lower back. Breathe in as you bring your legs up and breathe out as you slowly pull your knees towards your chest. Continue to breathe deeply as you hold your knees in a comfortable position.

Back Diary

Use the following pages weekly to record changes, activities and events as you work to improve and strengthen your back. A personal record of your exercise program and the process of physical change which results can be valuable information. This diary can make you more conscious about changes that occur over a period of time, and serve as a source of inspiration for continuing to take your health into your own hands.

Your weekly back account will tell you:
- where your pain focuses and radiates.
- when your back hurts the most
- what causes your back problems
- what makes your back pain worse
- which techniques help relieve the pain

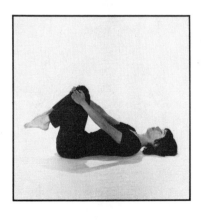 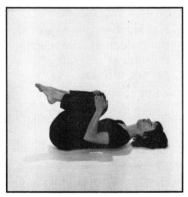

BACK DIARY
KEEPING TRACK OF MY BACK ACCOUNT

Date_____

Present condition of my back:

☐ painful   ☐ tense

☐ stiff   ☐ aching

☐ tired   ☐ _____

The pain is:

☐ sharp   ☐ off and on

☐ dull   ☐ steady

When my back hurts the most: _____ (time of day)

☐ after sleeping   ☐ during work

☐ before sleeping ☐ _____

Where my pain is centered:

Use the drawing provided.
Mark in color the area of most
discomfort.

Where the pain radiates:

Use another color to show how
the discomfort travels and to
illustrate other areas of tension,
pain or stiffness.

☐ up the upper back

☐ into the lower back

☐ into the neck

☐ through the ribs

☐ down the back of the leg

☐ along the side of the leg

☐ into the hips

☐ across the back

What makes my back worse:

- ☐ standing
- ☐ sitting
- ☐ bending
- ☐ lifting
- ☐ driving

- ☐ cold weather
- ☐ menstruation
- ☐ stress
- ☐ constipation
- ☐ pressure from:

_____

My back discomfort has affected my:

- ☐ sleep
- ☐ breathing
- ☐ outlook on life
- ☐ relationships

- ☐ appetite
- ☐ elimination
- ☐ work

Describe any changes of feeling you are experiencing as a result.

_____

_____

_____

What has helped to relieve my back pain?

- ☐ massage
- ☐ meditation
- ☐ Acu-Yoga exercises
  (specify:_____

- ☐ sleep
- ☐ pressure points
- ☐ exercise (specify kind,
  i.e. swimming, etc.)

_____   _____

PRACTICE: Choose 3 techniques or exercises from this book.

1. _____ on page _____
2. _____ on page _____
3. _____ on page _____

RESULTS: Describe the changes that have occurred in your back.

_____

_____

_____

_____

_____

_____

_____

BACK DIARY
KEEPING TRACK OF MY BACK ACCOUNT

Date_____

Present condition of my back:

☐ painful   ☐ tense

☐ stiff   ☐ aching

☐ tired   ☐ _____

The pain is:

☐ sharp   ☐ off and on

☐ dull   ☐ steady

When my back hurts the most: _____(time of day)

☐ after sleeping   ☐ during work

☐ before sleeping ☐ _____

Where my pain is centered:

Use the drawing provided.
Mark in color the area of most
discomfort.

Where the pain radiates:

Use another color to show how
the discomfort travels and to
illustrate other areas of tension,
pain or stiffness.

☐ up the upper back

☐ into the lower back

☐ into the neck

☐ through the ribs

☐ down the back of the leg

☐ along the side of the leg

☐ into the hips

☐ across the back

What makes my back worse:
- ☐ standing
- ☐ sitting
- ☐ bending
- ☐ lifting
- ☐ driving
- ☐ cold weather
- ☐ menstruation
- ☐ stress
- ☐ constipation
- ☐ pressure from:

_____

My back discomfort has affected my:
- ☐ sleep
- ☐ breathing
- ☐ outlook on life
- ☐ relationships
- ☐ appetite
- ☐ elimination
- ☐ work

Describe any changes of feeling you are experiencing as a result.

_____
_____
_____

What has helped to relieve my back pain?
- ☐ massage
- ☐ meditation
- ☐ Acu-Yoga exercises
  (specify:_____
- ☐ sleep
- ☐ pressure points
- ☐ exercise (specify kind,
  i.e. swimming, etc.)

_____   _____

PRACTICE: Choose 3 techniques or exercises from this book.
1. _____ on page _____
2. _____ on page _____
3. _____ on page _____

RESULTS: Describe the changes that have occurred in your back.

_____
_____
_____
_____
_____
_____
_____

BACK DIARY
KEEPING TRACK OF MY BACK ACCOUNT

Date_____

Present condition of my back:

☐ painful   ☐ tense

☐ stiff   ☐ aching

☐ tired   ☐ _____

The pain is:

☐ sharp   ☐ off and on

☐ dull   ☐ steady

When my back hurts the most: _____(time of day)

☐ after sleeping   ☐ during work

☐ before sleeping   ☐ _____

Where my pain is centered:

Use the drawing provided.
Mark in color the area of most
discomfort.

Where the pain radiates:

Use another color to show how
the discomfort travels and to
illustrate other areas of tension,
pain or stiffness.

☐ up the upper back

☐ into the lower back

☐ into the neck

☐ through the ribs

☐ down the back of the leg

☐ along the side of the leg

☐ into the hips

☐ across the back

What makes my back worse:

- ☐ standing
- ☐ sitting
- ☐ bending
- ☐ lifting
- ☐ driving

- ☐ cold weather
- ☐ menstruation
- ☐ stress
- ☐ constipation
- ☐ pressure from:

_____

My back discomfort has affected my:

- ☐ sleep
- ☐ breathing
- ☐ outlook on life
- ☐ relationships

- ☐ appetite
- ☐ elimination
- ☐ work

Describe any changes of feeling you are experiencing as a result.

_____

_____

_____

What has helped to relieve my back pain?

- ☐ massage
- ☐ meditation
- ☐ Acu-Yoga exercises
  (specify:_____

- ☐ sleep
- ☐ pressure points
- ☐ exercise (specify kind,
  i.e. swimming, etc.)

_____   _____

PRACTICE: Choose 3 techniques or exercises from this book.

1. _____ on page _____
2. _____ on page _____
3. _____ on page _____

RESULTS: Describe the changes that have occurred in your back.

_____

_____

_____

_____

_____

_____

_____

BACK DIARY
KEEPING TRACK OF MY BACK ACCOUNT

Date_____

Present condition of my back:

☐ painful   ☐ tense

☐ stiff   ☐ aching

☐ tired   ☐ _____

The pain is:

☐ sharp   ☐ off and on

☐ dull   ☐ steady

When my back hurts the most: _____(time of day)

☐ after sleeping   ☐ during work

☐ before sleeping ☐ _____

Where my pain is centered:

Use the drawing provided.
Mark in color the area of most
discomfort.

Where the pain radiates:

Use another color to show how
the discomfort travels and to
illustrate other areas of tension,
pain or stiffness.

☐ up the upper back

☐ into the lower back

☐ into the neck

☐ through the ribs

☐ down the back of the leg

☐ along the side of the leg

☐ into the hips

☐ across the back

116.

What makes my back worse:
- ☐ standing
- ☐ sitting
- ☐ bending
- ☐ lifting
- ☐ driving
- ☐ cold weather
- ☐ menstruation
- ☐ stress
- ☐ constipation
- ☐ pressure from:

_____

My back discomfort has affected my:
- ☐ sleep
- ☐ breathing
- ☐ outlook on life
- ☐ relationships
- ☐ appetite
- ☐ elimination
- ☐ work

Describe any changes of feeling you are experiencing as a result.

_____

_____

_____

What has helped to relieve my back pain?
- ☐ massage
- ☐ meditation
- ☐ Acu-Yoga exercises
  (specify:_____
- ☐ sleep
- ☐ pressure points
- ☐ exercise (specify kind,
  i.e. swimming, etc.)

_____   _____

PRACTICE: Choose 3 techniques or exercises from this book.

1. _____ on page _____
2. _____ on page _____
3. _____ on page _____

RESULTS: Describe the changes that have occurred in your back.

_____

_____

_____

_____

_____

_____

_____

_____

117.

BACK DIARY
KEEPING TRACK OF MY BACK ACCOUNT

Date_____

Present condition of my back:

☐ painful   ☐ tense

☐ stiff   ☐ aching

☐ tired   ☐ _____

The pain is:

☐ sharp   ☐ off and on

☐ dull   ☐ steady

When my back hurts the most: _____(time of day)

☐ after sleeping   ☐ during work

☐ before sleeping   ☐ _____

Where my pain is centered:

Use the drawing provided.
Mark in color the area of most
discomfort.

Where the pain radiates:

Use another color to show how
the discomfort travels and to
illustrate other areas of tension,
pain or stiffness.

☐ up the upper back

☐ into the lower back

☐ into the neck

☐ through the ribs

☐ down the back of the leg

☐ along the side of the leg

☐ into the hips

☐ across the back

What makes my back worse:
- ☐ standing
- ☐ sitting
- ☐ bending
- ☐ lifting
- ☐ driving
- ☐ cold weather
- ☐ menstruation
- ☐ stress
- ☐ constipation
- ☐ pressure from:

_____

My back discomfort has affected my:
- ☐ sleep
- ☐ breathing
- ☐ outlook on life
- ☐ relationships
- ☐ appetite
- ☐ elimination
- ☐ work

Describe any changes of feeling you are experiencing as a result.

_____

_____

_____

What has helped to relieve my back pain?
- ☐ massage
- ☐ meditation
- ☐ Acu-Yoga exercises (specify:_____
- ☐ sleep
- ☐ pressure points
- ☐ exercise (specify kind, i.e. swimming, etc.)

_____   _____

PRACTICE: Choose 3 techniques or exercises from this book.

1. _____ on page _____
2. _____ on page _____
3. _____ on page _____

RESULTS: Describe the changes that have occurred in your back.

_____

_____

_____

_____

_____

_____

_____

_____

BACK DIARY
KEEPING TRACK OF MY BACK ACCOUNT

Date_____

Present condition of my back:

☐ painful   ☐ tense

☐ stiff   ☐ aching

☐ tired   ☐ _____

The pain is:

☐ sharp   ☐ off and on

☐ dull   ☐ steady

When my back hurts the most: _____(time of day)

☐ after sleeping ☐ during work

☐ before sleeping ☐ _____

Where my pain is centered:

Use the drawing provided.
Mark in color the area of most
discomfort.

Where the pain radiates:

Use another color to show how
the discomfort travels and to
illustrate other areas of tension,
pain or stiffness.

☐ up the upper back

☐ into the lower back

☐ into the neck

☐ through the ribs

☐ down the back of the leg

☐ along the side of the leg

☐ into the hips

☐ across the back

120.

What makes my back worse:

☐ standing   ☐ cold weather
☐ sitting   ☐ menstruation
☐ bending   ☐ stress
☐ lifting   ☐ constipation
☐ driving   ☐ pressure from:

_____

My back discomfort has affected my:

☐ sleep   ☐ appetite
☐ breathing   ☐ elimination
☐ outlook on life   ☐ work
☐ relationships

Describe any changes of feeling you are experiencing as a result.

_____
_____
_____

What has helped to relieve my back pain?

☐ massage   ☐ sleep
☐ meditation   ☐ pressure points
☐ Acu-Yoga exercises ☐ exercise (specify kind,
   (specify:_____)   i.e. swimming, etc.)

_____   _____

PRACTICE: Choose 3 techniques or exercises from this book.

1._____ on page _____
2._____ on page _____
3._____ on page _____

RESULTS: Describe the changes that have occurred in your back.

_____
_____
_____
_____
_____
_____
_____
_____

Glossary

Acupressure: A method of bodywork that uses the Chinese system of Acupuncture points and meridians combined with Japanese finger pressure techniques to release muscular tensions and increase circulation.

Acupuncture: A traditional method of Chinese medicine in which fine needles are inserted into the body in key points to release internal blockages and balance energy.

Acu-Yoga: An integration of Acupressure and Yoga used for self-treatment.

Adjustment: A Chiropractic manipulation to properly align the vertebrae of the spinal column.

Affirmations: Personal statements said aloud or thought to oneself that positively validate different aspects of one's existence. They are used to visualize and increase the benefits of Acu-Yoga techniques.

Alignment: Having the spinal vertebrae in proper line.

Blockage: An accumulation or congestion of energy in or surrounding an Acupressure point. Blockages in a meridian may ache, be painful, or feel numb before manifesting as a physical symptom.

Breathing Awareness: The ability to deepen and direct the breath into different parts of the body through concentration and relaxation.

Centering: The process of gaining awareness of the mind and body. This enables a person to be more conscious in the present moment.

Cervical Vertebrae: The seven spinal bones of the neck: see diagram, page 39.

Chi: A Chinese word for vital energy. It has been translated as "material energy" or "vital matter" which circulates through the meridians.

Chronic Muscular Tension: A long term condition in which the muscle fibers are held indefinitely in a shortened, contracted state.

Coccyx: The tailbone; see diagram, page 39.

Deep Relaxation: The letting go of all parts of the body and mind to allow a natural flow of energy to circulate in its natural course. To completely relax after strenuous exercise is the best way to recharge the nervous system.

Disease: An imbalance in the system as a whole.

Distal Points: Acupressure points located a distance from the area they benefit: see Local Points.

Energy: The basis of all forms of life and matter in the universe. It is a dynamic force that circulates through the body in specific pathways called meridians.

Energy Blockage: An obstruction to the free flow of vital matter which manifests physically as tension, pain, or stiffness. Thoughts and emotions can also cause energy blockages.

Frontal Points: Acupressure points located on the front of the body.

Holistic: An approach to life based on a perspective that all forms of existence are unified, that the whole equals more than the sum of its parts and that every aspect, whether internal or external, affects the whole.

Homeostatic: A mechanism of equilibrium or balance.

Hypertension: Abnormally high arterial blood pressure.

Impotence: The inability to have satisfying sexual relationships. Unusual vaginal discharge or premature ejaculation can be preliminary signs of developing impotence.

Jin Shin: A highly developed Acupressure massage technique which uses gentle-to-deep finger pressure applied to specific points on the human anatomy. This system releases tension and rebalances all areas of the body.

Ki: The Japanese word for the vital life energy which concentrates in all living things. It circulates through the human body in pathways called meridians.

Life Force: The vital energy contained in all things. The three main types are:
(1) the energy that circulates through the body via the meridians.
(2) the power generated from the human qualities of love, devotion, determination, will power and positive thinking or projection; and
(3) the forces of nature which include the wind, rain, sun, heat, magnetism, gravity, and electricity.

Local Points: Acupressure Points located in the area that they benefit: see Distal Points.

Lumbar Vertebrae: The last five spinal bones above the sacrum, on the lower back.

Lumbosacral Area: Area of the lower back where the lumbar vertebrae join the sacrum.

Medial: Towards the center of the body.

Meditation: Focussing one's attention for developing the spiritual capabilities of the mind.

Meridians: The pathways along which Ki energy flows through the body, connecting the various Acupressure/Acupuncture points and the internal organs.

Yin Meridians		Yang Meridians	
Lung	Lu	Large Intestine	LI
Spleen	Sp	Stomach	St
Heart	H	Small Intestine	SI
Kidney	K	Bladder	B
Triple Warmer	TW	Pericardium	P
Liver	Lv	Gall Bladder	GB
Conception Vessel	CV	Governing Vessel	GV

Metatarsals: The bones between the ankle and toes, on the top of the foot.

Movement Therapy: Utilizing dance and creative movements as a form of self healing.

Nervous System: The network of nerves which regulates muscular functioning. It influences the coordination of every cell, organ, and system in the body.

Pressure points: Places on the human anatomy with high levels of electrical conductivity. They tend to be located in neuro-muscular junctions, in the joints, or where bones lies close to the skin along a meridian.

Referred Pain: Pain generated in one area of the body but felt in another.

Sacral: Having to do with the sacrum.

Sacrum: The flat triangular bone in the lower back located at the base of the spine; see diagram, page 39.

Sacroilliac Joints: The 2 places in the lower back where the sacrum joins the hip bones.

Shiatsu: A Japanese form of Acupressure which uses various finger pressure massage techniques on points along the meridians.

Solar Plexus: A large network of nerves that join at the upper abdomen.

Spinal Column: The backbone, composed of a series of bones called vertebrae, which are stacked on top of one another; it protects the spinal cord.

Spinal Cord: The thick cord of nerve tissue of the central nervous system that runs through the spinal column and into the brain.

Spinal Discs: The layer of fibrous connective tissue with small masses of cartilage located between each vertebrae.

Spinal Vertebrae: see Vertebrae.

Thoracic Vertebrae: The twelve spinal vertebrae, below the neck, in the upper and middle back; see diagram, page 39.

Vertebrae: The bones of the spinal column through which runs the spinal cord; see Cervical, Thoracic, and Lumbar Vertebrae.

Visualization: A creative process of forming images and thoughts which positively directs one's life.

Yin and Yang: The two polar forces which interact on all levels of existence, creating constant change.

> Yang — is the active or contractive force
> Yin — is the passive or expansive force

BIBLIOGRAPHY

Academy of Traditional Chinese Medicine. *An Outline of Chinese Acupuncture.* Peking: Foreign Languages Press, 1975.

Brena, Steven F., M.D. *Yoga and Medicine.* New York, New York: Penguin Books, 1973.

Brown, Isadore. "Intensive Exercises for the Lower Back," *Physical Therapy.* Vol. 50, No. 4, April, 1970.

Chamberlain, Godfrey. "Backache II," *British Medical Journal.* April, 1971.

Finneson, Bernard and Freese, Arthur. *The New Approach to Low Back Pain.* Berkeley Publishing Corp., 1975.

Gach, Michael Reed. *Acu-Yoga: Self-Help Techniques.* Tokyo, Japan: Japan Publications, 1981.

Garde, Raghanath K., M.D. *Principles and Practice of Yoga Therapy.* Lakemont, Georgia: Tarnhelm, 1970.

Kraus, Hans. "Prevention of Low Back Pain," *Journal of Occupational Medicine.* November, 1967.

Lettvin, Maggie. *Maggie's Back Book.* Houghton Mifflin, 1976.

Mann, Felix. *Atlas of Acupuncture.* Philadelphia, Pennsylvania: International Ideas, 1970.

Masunaga, Shizuto. *Zen Shiatsu.* Tokyo, Japan: Japan Publications, 1977.

Root, Leon, M.D. and Kierman, Thomas. *Oh, My Aching Back.* Signet, 1973.

Serizawa, Katsusuke, M.D. Massage: *The Oriental Method; Tsubo: Vital Points for Oriental Therapy.* Tokyo, Japan: Japan Publications, 1976.

Simons, Gene and Mirabile, Matthew. "An Analysis and Interpretation of Industrial Medical Data: With Concentration on Back Problems," *Journal of Occupational Medicine*. Vol. 14, No. 3, March, 1972.

Smith, Clyde F. "Physical Management of Muscular Lower Back Pain," *Canadian Medical Assoc. Journal*. Vol. 117, No. 6, September 17, 1977.

Tauber, Joseph. "An Unorthodox Look at Backaches," *Journal of Occupational Medicine*. Vol. 12, April, 1970.

Teeguarden, Iona. *Acupressure Way of Health*. Japan: Japan Publications, 1978.

Todd, Mabel Elsworth. *The Thinking Body*. New York, New York: Dance Horizons Republications, 1975.

Index

buttock pain, 86, *see also* sciatica, pregnancy and menstruation

C

calcium and menstrual cramps, 68
calcium deposits, 100
calf, spasms or tightness in, 57
cardiac pains, 45, 46, 62
cardiovascular problems, 62
Cat Cow exercise, 33
causes of back pain, 11
cerebrospinal fluid, 41, Glossary
cervical vertebrae—*see* neck, vertebrae, and Glossary
Chair Exercises, 47-51, 59
chest pain, 62, *see also* cardiac pains and cardiovascular problems
chills, resistance to, 46
chiropractic, 5, 15
circulation, 10, 15, 21, 40, 56, 59, 61, 62, 99, 101, 102, 103
clothing, restrictive, 13
Cobra Pose, 44
coccyx, 39, 102, and Glossary
cold, 61
cold feet, 41, 51, 57, 66
cold hands, 21, 22, 49, 61
colds, 45
colds, resistance to, 46
colitis, 45, 51, 64
complaining, 63
compresses, hot, 24, 27, 55, *see also* ginger compresses
constipation, 21, 48, 51, 57, 63, 64, 91
contractions—*see* muscle contractions
coordination, lack of, 61
coughing, 12
Couples, Exercises for, 89
cramps, 27, 57, *see also* menstrual tension
Custom Back Roller, 106

D

daily practice, 5, 14, 19, 47
depression, 21, 27, 46
diaphragm, 27, 28 *see also* breathing

diet—*see* appetite, digestive problems
diet and the lower back, 37
diet and menstruation, 68
digestive problems, 21, 27, 28, 41, 56, 63, *see also* appetite
disc, slipped, 88
discs—*see* spinal discs
distal points, 27, 51, 88
dizziness, 56
Dollar Pose, 34, 48
dysmenorrhea (pain with menstruation), 67, *see also* pregnancy and menstruation

E

Ear Reflexology, 101
Elbow Lift, 49
emotional holding, 11
emotions, 20, 24, 27, 29, 56, 62
see also stress, anger, anxiety, apathy, depression, fear, grief, hysteria, melancholy, worry
endocrine system, 68, 99
endorphine, 10
exercise, 12, 15, 37
exercise principles, 14
Exercises for Couples, 89-93
eye problems, 45, 48, 61

F

fatigue, 31, 48, 49, 57, 61, 63
fear, 29, 45
feet—*see* foot
feet, cold, 41, 51, 57, 66
fever, 62
fever, resistance to, 46
first-aid Acupressure points, 55
Flattening the Lower Back, 32
flexibility of the back, 14-27, 29
flexibility of the spine, 11, 14, 19, 31, 39, 44, 55
flu, resistance to, 46
foot cramps, 66
foot pain, 57
Foot Reflexology, 101
forbidden points for pregnancy, 65
friendships, 92, *see also* Exercises for Couples
frustration, 27, 58, 61, 64

lumbar pain, 45
lumbar vertebrae—*see* lower back
vertebrae, and Glossary
lungs, 20, 37, 40, 62

M

marital problems, 92, *see also*
Exercises for Couples
massage—*see* Acupressure Massage
massage, internal, 23, 56
Master Back Point, 85
meditation, 56, 98-99, and Glossary
Meditation, breathing, 98
Meditation for Strengthening
the Spine, 99
meditation techniques, 99
melancholy, 62
menstrual tension, including
cramps, 64-68
menstruation, 66-68
menstruation, irregular, 45
meridians—*see* Acupressure
Meridians
mental pressures, 55
metabolic rate, 99
middle of the back, 27-35, 45, 46
48, 89, 90, 102
migraines, 21, *see also* headache
mobility in the hip joint, 59
morning sickness, 65
muscle contractions, 13, 55
muscular cramps—*see* cramps
muscular spasms, 21, 27, 57, 62
muscular tension, 9, 10, 11, 13,
23, 103, 105

N

nausea, 56
Neck Press, exercise, 25-26, 50
neck stiffness, 21, 24, 45, 57, 61
neck tension and pain, 12, 21,
24-26, 45, 46, 49, 50, 55, 61, 102
nerves, 12, 15, 19, 27, 40, 44, 64,
97, 99, 100, 101
nerve endings, 56, 100
nervous disorders, 41
nervous system rejuvenation, 99
nervousness, 21, 34, 41, 44, 45,
50, 55, 56, 61, 68
neuralgia, 21, 62, 102

O

occupational disability, 5
organs—*see* internal organs
Oriental healing, 5, 9, 12, 29, 37
osteopathic adjustments, 5
overeating, 46, 48, 63
oxygenation of the blood—
see blood

P

pain, *see* ankle, arm, back,
buttock, cardiac, chest,
hip, knee, leg, neck, sciatica,
shoulder, thigh
"pain-gateway" theory, 10
painful walking, 58, 101
pancreas, 37
Pelvic Raise, exercise, 23
pelvic tension, 64, *see also* sciatica
perineum, perineal disorders, 67
physical therapy, 5
pituitary gland, 10
Plow Pose, 46
pneumonia, 62
posture, 5, 9, 11-12, 14, 15, 19,
29, 41, 46
pregnancy, 65-68
preventive measures for the back,
5, 32, 44, 97, *see also* healthy
back

R

recovery, accelerated, 56
referred pain, 12, and Glossary
Reflexology, 56, 66, 100-102
rejuvenate the back, 99
rejuvenate the body, 101
rejuvenate the nervous system, 99
relaxation, deep, 10, 14
Release, General Back, 81-82
Release, Lower Back, 83-85
reproductive problems—*see*
sexual-reproductive problems
resistance to illness, 46, 47
respiratory problems, 20, 27
rheumatism, 61
rhythm, 14
rigidity in the neck and back, 55
Rock and Roll, exercise, 35

S

sacral vertebrae—*see* sacrum, vertebra, Glossary

sacroilliac joint, 64, 102, and Glossary

sacrum, 45, 64, 67, and Glossary

salt intake, 29

scapula (shoulder blades), 102

sciatic nerve/sciatica, 12, 57, 58-60, 63, 64, 102

scoliosis, 12, 44

sedentary lives, 11

self-help, 15, 19, 20, 24, 38, 47, 58, 68, 100, 106

severe lower back pain, 36

sex-related hormones, 64

sexual activity, 29

sexual imbalances, 44

sexual-reproductive problems, 29, 33, 64, 91, *see also* impotency

Shiatsu, 6, 9, 57, 71-80, 104

shoulder blades—*see* scapula

shoulder tension, 22, 23, 45, 46, 47, 49, 61, 62, 102

sinus headache, 48

sneezing, 12

sleep, 11, 15

snoring, 28, 63

solar plexus, 27, 28, and Glossary

sore throat—*see* throat

spasms—*see* muscular spasms

speech problems, 45

spinal adjustment, 19, 32, *see also* spinal alignment, and Glossary

spinal alignment, 11, 12, 15, 19, 42, and Glossary

spinal column, 11, 14, 15, 39, 40, 102, and Glossary

spinal cord, 10, 12, 39, 40, 41, and Glossary

spinal curve, 11-12

Spinal Flex, exercise, 41

spinal discs, 12, 19, and Glossary

spinal flexibility—*see* flexibility of the spine

spinal movement, 5

spinal problems, 39-46

spinal twist(s), 42, 51, 59

spine, elongation of, 15

spleen, 27, 37, 40, 89

Spleen Meridian (Sp), 66

sterility, sexual, 64, *see also* sexual-reproductive problems

stiffness—*see* back, body, knee, leg, or neck stiffness

stomach, 27, 40, 63, *see also* abdomen

Stomach Meridian (St), 66

strength of the spine, 19

stress, 24, 29, 61, 62, 99, and Glossary

stretching, 5, 9, 14, 15, 19, 57, 104, *see also* Acu-Yoga Exercises

suicidal, 45

surgery, 5

T

tension, 20, 27, 92, *see also* abdominal, back, menstrual, muscular, neck, pelvic, and shoulder tensions

thigh pain—*see* sciatica

thighs tight, 57

thoracic vertebrae—*see* middle of the back, vertebrae, and Glossary

throat, sore, 50, 61

throat, swollen, 61

thyroid (conditions), 40, 46, 61

tools for relieving back pain, 105-107

toxins, removal of, 10

trauma of back injury, 55-56

treatment for others, 60, 71-93

U

upper back, 20-23, 34, 45, 46, 47, 62, 102

Upper Back Opener, exercise, 22, 47

uptightness, 46, 47, *see also* neck and shoulder problems

urinary problems, 51, 57, 63, 64, 91, *see also* bladder

uterus, 67

V

vaginal discharge, 45, 64, *see also* sexual-reproductive problems, menstruation and pregnancy

vaginal problems, 67

About the Author

MICHAEL REED GACH founded the Acupressure Workshop of Berkeley, California in 1976. As Director of the Workshop he teaches classes on various forms of Acupressure: Jin Shin, Shiatsu, Acupressure Massage, Reflexology, Dō-In, and Acu-Yoga. He originated Acu-Yoga, which is based on his own experience and research in Acupressure and Yoga. His current focus is on teaching Acupressure for stress management.

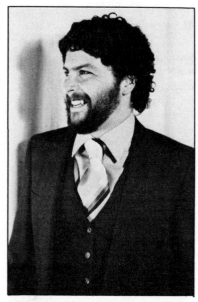

During the past five years Michael has led hundreds of classes, workshops, and seminars (locally and nationally) for various schools, centers, clinics, associations and colleges throughout the San Francisco Bay Area, and has developed a training program specifically for nurses and other health professionals. The Acupressure Workshop offers nurses Continuing Education credit for the courses he teaches.

Michael teaches classes to people in all walks of life throughout California and abroad. He is dedicated to helping people learn to help themselves and others in a holistic way, using safe and effective methods. Michael encourages people to be responsible for their health and improve the quality of their life by using Acupressure and Yoga, along with good nutrition, exercise, productive work and positive thinking. To obtain information about his activities and arrange workshops in other locations, contact the Acupressure Workshop, 1533 Shattuck Avenue, Berkeley, CA 94709.

The Acupressure Workshop offers a comprehensive,
150-hour certified training program
in Acupressure Massage.
The school is approved by the California State
Superintendent of Public Instructions,
Department of Education.

Also by Michael Reed Gach:

ACU-YOGA: Self-Help Techniques for Relieving Stress and Tension, ($12.95), Japan Publications, Inc. 1981, distributed by Bookpeople in Berkeley, CA and Harper & Row.

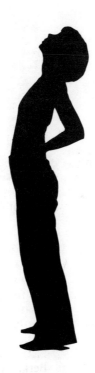

HEALTH AND BEAUTY are contingent upon the flexibility of the spine. If your spine is flexible and in alignment, the result can be seen in your whole body. If you have a limber spine you will have a youthful body; stiffness in the spine is a sign of aging. Beauty is a reflection of inner harmony and good health. Parts of the body not regularly used tend to contract as you grow older, and this rigidity is a slow form of atrophy. If a person, however, is well-balanced, gets enough exercise, and has a harmonious lifestyle, he or she will glow with the naturally beautiful inner radiance of vibrancy and health.   §

NOTES

BOOK & CASSETTE
Order Form

Please send me:

_____ Copies of the *Bum Back Book*
@ $7.95 plus $1.00 for handling & shipping, each

_____ Cassette Tape(s) of the *Bum Back Book* Exercises
@ $8.95 plus $1.00 for handling & shipping, each

_____ Copies of the *Acu-Yoga* book by Michael Reed Gach
@ $12.95 plus $1.00 for handling & shipping, each

_____ Cassette Tapes(s) of *Acu-Yoga* Exercises for the spine
@ $8.95 plus $1.00 for handling & shipping, each

_____ *Acupressure Flash Cards* illustrating 30 main points
@ $4.95 plus $1.00 for handling & shipping, each

_____ *Acupressure for Health Professionals*: Specific points for
common ailments, 28 pages.
@ $5.95 plus $1.00 for handling & shipping, each

_____ *Fundamentals of Acupressure*: Course booklet with two
cassette tapes narrated by Michael Reed Gach.
@ $18.95 plus $1.00 for handling & shipping, each

_____ List of recommended books

_____ Prices on color video tapes

California residents please add 6½% sales tax.
Orders of 10 or more of a single item receive a 20% discount.

Enclosed is $ _____ .

Name _____

Address _____

City & State _____ Zip _____

Send this form with your check or money order to:

AcuPress Publications

1533 Shattuck Ave. · Berkeley, CA 94709 · (415) 845-1059

Acupressure Training

Approved by the
Superintendent of Public Instruction,
California State Department of Education

This one month intensive (150-hour) training program, originated by Michael Reed Gach, offers a comprehensive study of various finger pressure point methods and natural health care practices. To receive further information, fill out the following form and send to the address below.

Please send:

_____ Brochure of Acupressure classes offered (free)

_____ School catalogue and application form(s) for the Acupressure Massage Certification program (free)

_____ Brochure(s) on the 1,000-hour Acupressure Therapy Program for professional practitioners and teacher training, $2 each

_____ Information on coordinating Acupressure Seminars and Workshops for groups of 20 or more people in my local area

I am interested in the following:

☐ Child Education   ☐ Psychology/Counseling
☐ Women's Health   ☐ Sports Medicine
☐ Bodywork   ☐ Stress Management
☐ Beauty (Spas, Salons)   ☐ Traditional Chinese Medicine
☐ Pain Management   ☐ Advanced Acupressure Techniques

☐ Other interests _____

Be specific about interests noted above: _____

_____

_____

Name _____

Address _____

City & State _____ Zip _____

Phone (Day) _____ (Evening) _____

Acupressure Institute

1533 Shattuck Ave. · Berkeley, CA 94709 · (415) 845-1059

MAY WE INTRODUCE YOU?

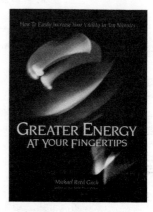

. . . to Michael Reed Gach's *Greater Energy At Your Fingertips*, a book that shows you how to increase your vitality easily in ten minutes using self-applied acupressure techniques. These easy-to-do self-help techniques enable you to maximize productivity throughout the day. Learn how to use posture, acupressure, and breathing techniques to rejuvenate your body and heighten your alertness. Over 150 photos show you not only how to boost your level of energy, but also how to reduce stress, sluggishness, fatigue, and how to relieve aches and pains, body tensions, headaches, and shoulder and neck tension.

Available at your local bookstore or directly from the publisher for $8.95 (plus 75¢ for Fourth Class postage or $2.25 for UPS fees; California residents please add 6.5% state sales tax to your order).

Send your order to: CELESTIAL ARTS, P.O. Box 7327, Berkeley, California 94707.

A WORD FROM CELESTIAL ARTS . . .

Celestial Arts is the publisher of many fine books on health, spirituality, personal growth, and psychology. For a copy of our free catalog, write or phone:

CELESTIAL ARTS
P.O. Box 7327
Berkeley, California 94707
(415) 524-1801